Pregnancy
sense

Meg Faure, Jacky Searle & Heather Wood

METZ PRESS

This book is dedicated to:

My daughters whose precious birth journey
I hope to share one day
Meg

My parents, Bob and Margaret –
thank you for everything
Jacky

The moms, dads and babies in my practice,
who inspire and nurture me more than they
could possibly know
Heather

Published by Metz Press
1 Cameronians Avenue
Welgemoed, 7530 South Africa

First published in 2016

Publisher: Wilsia Metz
Editor: Wilsia Metz
Designer: Liezl Maree
Illustratior: Nikki Miles
Proofreader: Lesley Hay-Whitton
Print production: Andrew de Kock
Printing and binding: Novus Print Solutions,
  Milnerton

ISBN 987-1-928201-87-8

With thanks to our colleagues and moms who
kindly contributed or proofread our work and
gave valuable feedback: Prof Lynette Denny
(foreword), psychologist Sheila Faure (emotional
content); paediatric dietician Kath Megaw (dietary
content); Tina Otte, Kate Christie, Lisa Raleigh,
moms in our community.

Authors' acknowledgements

Writing a book with two other exceptional clinicians is a bonding process. With over 60 years of combined experience, our knowledge and outlook was bound to be different. Yet, with one mission – to share the journey towards a safe, sensational and empowered birth – we connected and collaborated in a way that we hadn't fully anticipated.

Early on a Thursday morning, we met as a team in the coffee shop of Vincent Pallotti Hosptial and as we finished off, we shared briefly about each of our own births. Between us we had seven very different birth stories – home birth, water birth, difficult posterior presentation delivered naturally, emergency Caesar, and planned elective Caesars. Our birth stories were as rich as they were varied. In an instant there was a deep connection between us, a bond, an understanding. We were reminded of the significance of birth for a woman and in talking about it we acknowledged the power and importance of birth and giving birth.

Meg
It is with deep gratitude that I thank Jacky and Heather for joining me as the 'parents' of this book. Your depth of knowledge and absolute passion for pregnancy, birth and the families you touch are inspirational. Like a pregnancy, writing a book takes immense time and energy from our lives and families. Thank you Philip, for being my support and for always encouraging me in the work I do. You remain my rock. James, Alex and Em – my journey has been yours too, thank you for your love and understanding. I love you more than you can know. Thank you to Wilsia at Metz Press – like a midwife you nurture the birth of each Sense-series book – delivering them with care. My books are always safe in your hands. Thank you for the amazing work you do.

Heather
Thank you to Meg and Jacky for the privilege of working closely with you – my admiration only grows. To my mom, June Rogers (Sister Francis), in whose footsteps I have unwittingly followed and from whom I inherited the confidence that birth was safe and that I would birth well. Thank you to my husband, Pete, and children, Sian and Thomas, who love me and keep me humble. And special thanks to my clients, the moms and dads who let me into their lives, allowing me the privilege of sharing their vulnerable selves. My joy and passion is to watch them grow wings and fly, becoming confident parents who delight in their babies.

Jacky
Contributing to this book has, a little like pregnancy, been a incredible learning experience – from my initial reaction (never, I don't write, I don't have time) to the appreciation of the honour of being asked, and the bonding experience of working with Meg and Heather, my passionate and professional co-authors. I've learnt from them, laughed with them, and been nurtured by them when times got tough! However, I was correct about the time, and the slog involved. And that could only be managed with the support and tolerance of my family. My love and thanks to my husband Michael, who quietly enables me to do what I do. To my darling sons Nicholas and Gregory – who make mothering the best work of all – I love you.

I would also like to acknowledge my teachers, the colleagues and midwives alongside whom I have worked, and the women I've looked after, all who have moulded me into who I am.

Contents

Foreword

This latest offering for women and their health-care workers on the miraculous, often difficult and challenging experience of falling pregnant, maintaining pregnancy and delivering a healthy baby, is rich with practical and wise advice.

Over the centuries it has become evident that the prenatal, natal and postnatal experience of pregnancy may have a critical impact on the future lives of children and their families. Children who experience neglect, lack of attachment, lack of self-worth and/or are exposed to a toxic environment *in utero* (drugs, alcohol, high levels of stress, interpersonal violence) frequently display dysfunctional behaviour in later life.

This book brings into focus the need to understand the importance of pre- and postnatal life, that creating a safe and loving environment for mother, father, child and family is crucial to the successful development of the next generation. The authors have taken a holistic approach to pregnancy and birthing and have covered difficult areas from sexual activity, to how to ensure the father is integrated into the pregnancy and the care of the mother and the child. There are detailed explanations in all chapters for women and their significant others about the processes that are taking place during their pregnancies from an emotional, physical, psychological and spiritual perspective. It encourages women to take ownership of their bodies, to make birth plans that feel comfortable and realistic, where they can be held in a wholesome and mindful manner. It also emphasises the experience of the foetus and the neonate, and the critical importance of creating safety, love, and trust in the newborn.

Globally there are many anomalies in the management of pregnancy, from over-medicalisation in the western world where in some countries the Caesarean section rate is over 80 per cent, to poor countries where mothers die as a result of non-availability of surgical intervention. There are also widespread reports internationally of women being ill-treated in birthing facilities, resulting in severe trauma and often significant post-partum depression. Childbirth is quite simply miraculous and should be protected, held, respected and treated with the greatest dignity. This book does exactly that and provides a wealth of wise, sensible and caring advice to expectant mothers and their families.

Lynette Denny
(Chair and Professor, Obstetrics and Gynaecology, University of Cape Town, Groote Schuur Hospital)

Introduction

Pregnancy is a unique time in life. For you, your partner, your tiny developing baby and your extended family, this is a period of enormous significance.

For your **baby**, it is the time when her future becomes a possibility and the potential for the rest of her life is laid down. For an expectant **mother**, pregnancy signifies a complete shift in who you are – emotionally, physically and socially. Becoming a mother is the single biggest transition you will make in your life. For a father or partner and the extended **family**, pregnancy creates an altered state of mind. Thinking beyond the now and those you know there is a realisation that the destiny of your future and future generations lies miraculously within the human being you love.

Like a stone falling into water, pregnancy creates ripples of effect.

In the middle of the ripple is your new baby growing and developing within the uterus. This tiny life is affected by the decisions you make in pregnancy. Her path in life will, to an extent, be affected by your health, mind-set and situation during the nine-month period. In Chapter 1, we will look at the significance of pregnancy for your baby.

The first ripple surrounding your foetus is the environment in which she grows – the safe space of your body. Pregnancy has an enormous physical effect on you: your body will change dramatically over nine months and there will be many questions in your mind as you go along. You will need to care for yourself, as you are the incubator for your baby (see Chapter 2).

Surrounding the physical state of pregnancy is the third ripple – your emotional world. Pregnancy and 'becoming a mom' will alter your psyche – the way you feel and see yourself – forever. This is a life stage like no other – it is like the transformation of adolescence but this shift is fast-tracked into nine months – you will not emerge unchanged. Preparing for your emotional transition is covered in Chapter 3.

Finally, the effects of your new baby and this pregnancy, birth and post-partum period will alter the social circle around you – your partner, other children, parents and friends.

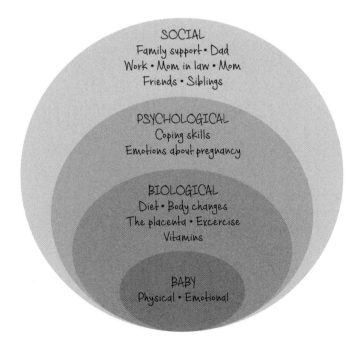

SOCIAL
Family support • Dad
Work • Mom in law • Mom
Friends • Siblings

PSYCHOLOGICAL
Coping skills
Emotions about pregnancy

BIOLOGICAL
Diet • Body changes
The placenta • Excercise
Vitamins

BABY
Physical • Emotional

Each of these ripples of effect will be looked at in a dedicated section of the book:

- **SECTION 1** covers the background information about the significance of pregnancy to your baby's development, your own growth and how your pregnancy will affect your relationships.
- **SECTION 2** looks at each stage of pregnancy – from falling pregnant to each month of the precious journey.
- **SECTION 3** looks at birth – preparing you for a sensational birth.
- **SECTION 4** covers the newborn days in terms of your and your baby's health.

By reading during your pregnancy you have already shown commitment to your baby. It is our hope that *Pregnancy sense* will empower you to parent with insight and flexibility. This is the secret to a sensible pregnancy and a sensational birth.

We also encourage you to visit our website, www.preggysense.com for further information, discussions and a full listing of resources.

CHAPTER 1

The sense behind pregnancy

Two blue lines! Pregnant! It feels surreal to Amanda. She and John have been dreaming of a baby but it has been a torturous journey. For seven years they tried every available fertility treatment before making the decision to stop trying to fall pregnant and to get off the emotional roller coaster.

This little life is a miracle for Amanda – the miracle of a child whom she thought she could not have – a natural conception against all odds.

Looking at her reflection in the bathroom mirror Amanda ponders the road ahead: Will this little one play hockey as she did? Will her child study quantum biology and embark on a trip to Mars, exploring the outer limits of human possibility? Will she walk down the aisle and have the joy of her own children one day?

As Amanda dreams of what the future may hold, she knows without doubt that these 9 months, 40 weeks, 280 days or 6 700 hours will have an impact on the rest of her child's life. No other period contains the potential to affect life in quite the same way.

Pregnancy is a nine-month magical passage of great significance, and preparing to have a baby is as wonderfully exciting as it is a weighty responsibility. Your ultimate goal is to provide your baby with the best start in life – a start that ensures she has the best chance at a full life. Pregnancy and birth affect your baby's physical health, her brain potential, the way she processes sensory information, her emotional happiness and, in fact, every facet of her life.

From conception until birth, over 6 700 hours, your baby forms on various levels:

- Genetically, your baby's blueprint for life will manifest.
- Physically, your baby's health – resistance to disease, predisposition to diabetes and obesity and many other aspects – will be shaped.
- Neurologically, your baby's brain will be prepared for all future development – physical coordination, intelligence, reasoning and creativity.
- Emotionally, the wiring of pathways that determine happiness, depression and engagement with other humans will begin to connect.

You have the chance to prepare the ingredients for your baby's life.

YOUR BABY'S BLUEPRINT

As Mom and Dad, you each provide half the genes that are the blueprint or script for your baby's life. These genes are the code you inherited from your own ancestors. This code determines hair colour, height and fingerprints. It programs potential genetic health issues and provides a platform for genius, musical brilliance or sporting prowess. It is the first ingredient for your child's future.

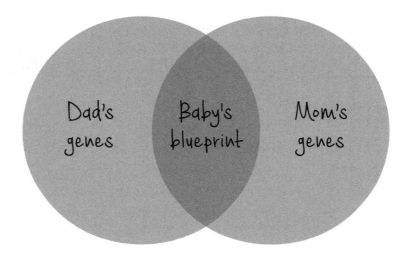

This blueprint is not a set mould; it is more like a script and a script is not cast in stone. *Romeo and Juliet* when performed in the Globe Theatre in the 1597 would have been very different from the 1996 version with Leonardo DiCaprio.

So it is with your baby – how her genes are expressed and played out in her personality and success in life is strongly influenced by the way you nurture her. More important than genes is whether your lifestyle is healthy, what relationships surround your baby and the society into which she is born. Your baby's future is greatly affected by how she is nurtured after conception – during pregnancy, in birth and in the time beyond birth. This is nurture – beyond the blueprint.

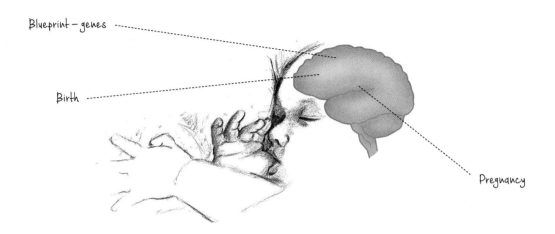

Blueprint — genes

Birth

Pregnancy

BEYOND THE BLUEPRINT

Pregnancy

Amanda had no idea she was pregnant. She had been feeling ill for a month and put it down to gastro. Discovering she is pregnant at 10 weeks means she has less than seven months of pregnancy ahead of her and she plans to make them count - providing the building blocks for her baby's development. This means a shift of diet, health and emotions.

Pregnancy is the first step in the building process; pregnancy provides the opportunity for each cell, including each vital neuron (brain cell), to end up in the right place, determining your baby's potential. During pregnancy, your baby develops all her senses, ready for birth and the first few years of life, when she will make sense of the world.

Brain development

In the first month of pregnancy, before you even know that you are pregnant, your baby's brain starts to develop. There are three essential parts to brain development:

1. In the first trimester, brain cells are *formed* deep in the centre of what will be the brain. During this early period of pregnancy, your baby cultivates around double the number of brain cells that she will need for life, and by birth she has 100 billion brain cells. Brain cells that are not needed or used will fall away over time.

2. Over the next few months of pregnancy, each brain cell *migrates* to the right place in the brain. It is this journey to a specific location that allows a brain cell to perform its designated function; for example, a visual brain cell needs to be in the right location to connect meaningfully to the visual pathways. The first trimester is a vulnerable time, when toxins and poor lifestyle choices can negatively affect the brain's architecture. As an example, alcohol consumption in pregnancy can affect your baby's brain cell migration.

3. Finally, from the second trimester onwards, the brain cells reach out and start to make *connections* (synapses) with each other — the brain is wired to connect. Between 20 weeks gestation and two years old, your baby's brain will make 15 000 connections per brain cell, enabling her to make sense of the world.

By the time Amanda finds out she is pregnant, her baby only weighs 10 g and yet 95 per cent of her organs are formed. It is a delicate period. What you eat, the alcohol you ingest, the stress you endure and how you feel in pregnancy all play a vital role, not only in refining the migration and connections of brain cells but also in the development of organs, thus affecting your baby's potential and providing the platform for future development.

Although babies are more resilient than we may think, it is wise to consider your choices if you are trying to fall pregnant or are pregnant as these early lifestyle choices may affect your little one.

Sensory development

By the end of the second trimester, all your baby's senses are developed, and in the third trimester she even starts to learn about her world.

- **Touch and proprioception**, the two body senses that give your baby feedback about her body, are the first senses to develop. Your baby will tend to **touch** the sensitive parts of her body (her face, mouth and hands) and ignore the parts that are less sensitive (her tummy) and the insensitive fontanel (which remains insensitive throughout pregnancy to allow for the impending squeeze through the birth canal). Moving against resistance in the tight uterine space gives **proprioceptive** feedback that tells her how to move after birth. It also introduces a sense of 'what's me and what's not', which develops in the first six months after birth.
- **Movement** (vestibular) sense is well developed by the third trimester and will be the sense that allows your little one to orient in response to gravity and turn head down – ready for birth.
- **Hearing** is well developed in the last trimester and is a sense that contributes to learning in pregnancy. By the end of pregnancy your baby will not only recognise your voice but also have a preference for her own mother tongue, recognising the language she will be spoken to after she is born.

> ## Making sense
> . . . .
> **Fontanel** refers to the soft spot on your baby's head where the skull bones have not yet fused. This closes as your baby's skull bones grow and by six weeks they usually meet.

This does not mean that we need to stimulate our babies *in utero*, though. Just being alive in this perfect uterine world provides the best possible stimulation for your little one.

Having your baby early

Since the uterine world is the perfect place for development to take place, premature births can have an effect on brain architecture and the way the blueprint manifests. It is not wise to **induce** natural labour or schedule a Caesarean section early, without good reason, as a full 40-week pregnancy in the ideal uterine environment is best for your baby.

If premature labour (before 37 weeks) is anticipated, you might be given corticosteroids to speed up maturity of the lungs and reduce the risk of other complications. In addition, it is wise to adjust the neonatal ICU environment to mimic the womb world. (See Chapter 16, p. 144 if you have a prem baby.)

GOOD FOR FOETAL DEVELOPMENT	RISKY FOR FOETAL DEVELOPMENT
• Good nutrition • Less stimulation • Happy emotions • Exercise • Rest • Full-term pregnancy	• Nutrient deficiency – retarded brain development and *spina bifida* • Drugs – stops transfer of nutrients and oxygen, affecting the brain • Alcohol – associated with faulty cell migration and brain cell death • Smoking – interferes with pruning and migration of neurons, and increases risk of prem baby • Certain infections, such as German measles • Sensory overstimulation • Toxic stress

Birth

Around 6 700 hours after conception you release your miracle to the world. Birth is the most powerful moment in a woman's life: a significant journey through pain to elation. Its significance will never leave you and it is vital that you empower yourself to make it your own, to do it your way and engage with all its joy. This book will help you understand birth in a way that will empower you to have a sensational birth.

YOU HAVE A SAY

Ultimately your method of labour, pain relief and birth should be a conscious and very personal choice. (Section 3 discusses your options for birth.) We live in a world where predictability and planning are the order of the day. For many women this order is extended into the birth process and they opt for a predictable process and the delivery of their baby via planned Caesarean section (C-section). For others, a more natural and baby driven approach is the preference. It is important to know that birth does not have to be a medicalised process – dictated by a medical system – and that ideally a balance should exist between your preference, your caregiver and your baby's needs.

YOUR BABY HAS SOME SAY

Regardless of your eventual choice of birth option (Caesarean section, water birth, natural delivery or any other method), it is important to recognise your baby's role in the birth process too. Babies determine the moment that labour begins and, to a degree, will influence the length of labour and method of delivery.

THE ILLUSION OF CHOICE

Reading this book you will become informed about birth and may find yourself having strong preferences. When you make these choices it is important that you are aware of the illusion of choice that you will be subject to. In a typical South African antenatal class, around three out of four women indicate they want a vaginal delivery; in reality three out of four will have a Caesarean section. The reason is twofold:

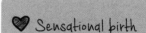

♡ Sensational birth
. . . .
It does not matter if you give birth naturally or with surgical assistance. What does matter is that you are empowered to make decisions and engage with your birth process and that you and your baby are healthy – the product of a unique blueprint, a healthy pregnancy and an informed and safe birth. This is the best start for a human life.

Birth is unpredictable

While you may feel that you have the ultimate say, the truth is that birth is unpredictable. Your focus should not be on a set method of birthing but on understanding birth options and being active and engaged in the process and choices. If you make this your focus and not an actual birth plan, you will have a sensational birth.

Choice of caregiver

Ultimately, your birth experience – how you labour and what pain relief you have and whether you end up having a C-section or natural birth – will also be strongly influenced by your choice of caregiver and whether you access private or state medical facilities. The message is: be empowered to understand your options and to choose your caregiver with consideration for the outcome you want (see p. 45).

The first day

The transition from womb to world is a challenging process for Baby and Mom. For your little one, there are enormous physical changes. Her blood flow through her heart changes direction as she takes her first breath. The hole in her heart closes to allow for effective pumping of blood to the body. Her temperature and breathing need to be self-regulated.

On a sensory level, the world is a very different space from the nurturing world of the womb she knows well. It is cold and bright, with a multitude of new sensations, such as hunger, the sensation of a nappy, and a Vitamin K injection.

This first day is important for latching and breast-feeding as well as for connecting with your little one. Latching may require help as it's a new skill for Mom and Baby. Chapter 17 will take you through the first day with your baby and look at breast-feeding in detail.

In an ideal world all babies, whether born by Caesarean section or normal vaginal delivery, do best when placed naked on their mother's naked chest after birth. This skin-to-skin contact or Kangaroo Mother Care (KMC) is very beneficial on a sensory, feeding and emotional level.

If your baby is ill or in distress after birth, or if you had a tough time in birth, your baby may be separated from you. This does not necessarily signify a break in bond or have long-term negative consequences – you need to do what is best for your baby under the circumstances.

The first six weeks

The transition from womb to world does not end on day one. The next six weeks are often a period of great shift for you – hormonally, emotionally and physically – and also for your baby. This transition lays down the path for the months ahead. Adjusting your baby's sensory world, and helping her to regulate her mood, sleep and feeding, is vital and is a steep learning curve.

KEEPING PERSPECTIVE

Carrying this miracle baby leaves Amanda feeling more than a little anxious. She is fearful of something going wrong and at times she also feels overwhelmed by the responsibility. Having no inkling that she was pregnant for the first 10 weeks, she had not limited her alcohol intake and was not on folic acid. Her mind is preoccupied with what she is already doing wrong as a mom.

These emotions are normal. Knowing the science of how a baby develops and the significance of pregnancy does allow you to make conscious choices about your life and the way you nurture your baby, but it is vital to keep perspective.

In pregnancy, birth and life:

- there will be things you can control and decisions you can make – this knowledge should empower you to make the right choices for you and your baby;
- there will be things you cannot control or have a say in and, while these aspects may leave you feeling disempowered and helpless, it is vital to put them in a box filled with acceptance and move on. Babies are very resilient; in fact, certain challenges and the way they are dealt with increase resilience and self-regulation. Don't despair when things are not perfect or don't go according to plan. Find a way to accept the things you cannot control.

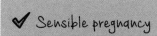

✔ Sensible pregnancy

Your baby is unlikely to be affected by your diet and lifestyle before you know you are pregnant as the placenta is not functional at this time, so there is less risk of transfer of teratogens from you to your baby before six and a half weeks of pregnancy.

The esSense of pregnancy

- 🌱 Your baby has the genetic blueprint for her development for life but it is not cast in stone – pregnancy, birth and the early years strongly affect your baby's potential.

- 🌱 The womb is the best place for your baby on a sensory and physical level. Premature birth and early induction of birth will have an impact on this.

- 🌱 Your lifestyle, emotions and choices in pregnancy and birth will have long lasting ramifications – it's only nine months – make it count.

- 🌱 The sensory world of the womb is ideal. An attitude of 'less is more' is true for the womb – there is no need to provide sensory stimulation for your baby *in utero* in any way.

- 🌱 It is essential to keep perspective – have a say and make your choices carefully when you can, but be flexible because in pregnancy, birth and life there will be aspects that simply don't go to plan. And that's okay for your baby.

CHAPTER 2

Your changing body

As a dancer, Sindi has always been a healthy person – more than just a passing fad, exercise and looking after her body have been a way of life. She is delighted to be pregnant but is finding that the changes to her body are throwing her out. She did not anticipate the morning sickness and fatigue of the early weeks. And, just as things started to improve, the hunger and weight gain kicked in. Like many women, Sindi is experiencing a hyper focus on her aches and pains and the so-called normal niggles of pregnancy.

As you embark on this journey, your baby is not the only one developing and transforming rapidly. You, too, will emerge from the process a new person. Your body will never be the same and for the foreseeable future (even beyond pregnancy) will no longer be your own.

YOUR BODY

From the moment of conception, when the egg is fertilised, hormones are released that orchestrate incredible changes in your body to accommodate and nourish your baby until birth, and enable you to feed your baby afterwards.

A miracle of life

Over and above the self-sacrifice and emotional shift of becoming a mother, the physical adaptations that make childbirth and breast-feeding possible are nothing short of a medical miracle. There are changes in your hormones (endocrinological changes), the structure of your body (anatomical changes) and the functions within your body (physiological changes). Your body anticipates the future needs of your baby and prepares for these very early in pregnancy, long before the foetus needs them. This is the miracle of pregnancy.

YOUR BODY DOESN'T REJECT YOUR BABY

Our bodies are built to fight and reject anything foreign that penetrates our body barriers. It is miraculous that you do not reject the foetus and placenta, which are genetically different from you. Pregnancy is the only time when the human body tolerates a tissue that is different from its own without complications. Early on in pregnancy, the placenta forms an 'immunologically privileged site'. As the placenta forms, genes responsible for attracting immune cells are switched off. Adjustments in the immune response in pregnancy allow your baby to form within your body.

HORMONES PROTECT THE PREGNANCY EARLY ON

In a normal menstrual cycle, after the release of an egg, the follicle that produces the egg in the ovary forms a *corpus luteum*. If the egg is fertilised, it starts to release human chorionic gonadotrophin (hCG), a hormone that maintains the *corpus luteum* in early pregnancy. The *corpus luteum* enlarges rapidly, producing the essential hormones of pregnancy until the 10th week, when the placenta takes over hormone production.

THE PLACENTA – A WHOLE NEW ORGAN

The placenta forms the interface between you and your baby, which is one of the biggest miracles of pregnancy. The foetal part of the placenta buries into the wall of the uterus, invades the surrounding tissue and comes into contact with your blood vessels. The placenta is an entirely new organ in your body, attached to the lining of your womb.

The placenta keeps your blood and your baby's blood supply separate, which is why you and your baby can have different blood types. At the same time it allows for the seamless exchange of nutrients, oxygen, antibodies, hormones and waste products. It filters certain toxins that could harm your baby and is a major producer of hormones that are important to maintain the pregnancy. In early pregnancy the placenta itself produces nutrients for the embryo.

THE ULTIMATE INCUBATOR

Your uterus grows from its non-pregnant size – that of a small pear, approximately 7,5 × 5 × 2,5 cm in size, with a capacity of 4 mℓ – to a structure measuring 28 × 24 × 21 cm and weighing 900 g with a capacity of 4 ℓ. The uterus changes shape as it grows, elongating and moving out of the pelvis and into the abdomen. The wall becomes thinner, and the supporting ligaments stretch. The muscle fibres prepare to contract, and the first Braxton Hicks contractions may occur by the end of the first trimester.

The opening of the uterus is the **cervix**. It performs two vital and contrasting functions in pregnancy. It must stay tightly closed to contain your baby for the duration of pregnancy, and then dilate in labour to allow the passage of a newborn baby. The mucus produced from glands in the cervix is thick and forms the mucous plug – an important barrier against infection.

During birth, the **vulva and vagina** need to stretch to a much greater capacity than ever before. During pregnancy there is a significant increase in blood supply and an increase in the size and number of muscle fibres. The connective tissue becomes looser. In addition, to protect your baby, the normal vaginal discharge becomes more acidic, keeping abnormal bacteria at bay.

A HOTHOUSE OF HORMONES

The foetus, ovaries and the placenta produce hormones important in pregnancy, labour and breast-feeding. These hormones include:

- **hCG** signals to the *corpus luteum* of the ovary to start producing oestrogen and progesterone to make your early pregnancy secure. hCG also plays a role in immunological tolerance, preventing your body from rejecting your baby as 'foreign'.
- **Relaxin** relaxes muscles and soft tissue, preventing contractions during pregnancy, and allowing softening of ligaments and joints, which is needed to create flexibility in your pelvis for your baby's birth.
- **Prolactin** plays a role in maintaining fluids and electrolytes in the foetus and amniotic fluid, and promotes uterine contractions. Together with oestrogen and progesterone, it stimulates the growth and development of your breasts, and its important function is the stimulation of breast milk production after birth.
- **Oestrogen**, released in large amounts, is responsible for growth of the uterus, ducts in your breasts and new blood vessels in the uterus and genital tract. It manages water and sodium levels, which contributes to water retention. It changes the connective tissue, allowing your skin to stretch and your cervix to open when the time comes.
- **Progesterone** balances the action of oestrogen in pregnancy. Initially it is responsible for the change in the lining of the uterus, preparing it for pregnancy, as well as altering the cervical mucus preventing further penetration by sperm. Progesterone prepares your breasts for breast-feeding and relaxes the muscle of

the uterus, inhibiting early labour. At the same time, it relaxes the digestive system and your blood vessels, contributing to bloating and constipation and sometimes causing varicose veins. It increases thirst, appetite and fat deposition.

BREASTS PREPARE TO FEED

The earliest signs of pregnancy often occur in the breasts in the form of tingling, tenderness and obvious blue veins beneath the skin. Your breasts will increase in size (by one to two cup sizes during pregnancy) as a result of an increased number of glands and ducts and deposits of fat. Your nipples enlarge and may become darker. Colostrum, the first breast milk, forms during pregnancy. You might not be aware of any colostrum or may simply see the dried granules on your nipple, or there might be leakage of colostrum by the third trimester.

> ### Making sense
> . . . .
> **Colostrum** is early breast milk produced in the last trimester of pregnancy and the first three days after your baby is born. Colostrum is rich in antibodies and protein, and sustains your baby until your milk comes in.

YOUR HEART AND BLOOD CHANGES

Your body produces 40 per cent more blood in pregnancy and your heart has to work much harder to pump it through your body. To do this, your heart rate increases by approximately 10 beats per minute and your blood vessels dilate, dropping your blood pressure. By 36 weeks your blood pressure rises again to pre-pregnancy levels. If your blood pressure becomes abnormally high, you need to be checked for preeclampsia and other causes of hypertension.

> ### Making sense
> . . . .
> **Preeclampsia**, also known as toxaemia or gestational proteinuric hypertension (GPH), is a complication of pregnancy identified by raised blood pressure and protein in the urine. Symptoms include headaches, unusual swelling and visual disturbances. It has potentially life-threatening consequences, needs specialist management and may be reason to deliver your baby early.

YOU BREATHE MORE EFFICIENTLY

Your growing baby pushes up your diaphragm and your ribcage moves outwards. While this may leave you feeling short of breath, you are actually more efficient at breathing and your oxygen consumption improves. You may find your breathing rate increases, especially after moderate exercise.

YOUR APPETITE AND DIGESTION SHIFT

In the first trimester, you may experience nausea and vomiting (morning sickness) owing to hormonal changes. This should resolve by 14 to 16 weeks, when thirst and appetite increase to cater for your growing baby's needs. There is general relaxation and slowing down of the gastrointestinal tract so that you can absorb more nutrients from your food. This may lead to bloating, flatulence and constipation.

Reflux of the acid contents of the stomach back into the oesophagus causes heartburn.

CLEARING OUT THE WASTE

Your kidneys have the vital role of processing waste. Since this is so essential in pregnancy, there is increased blood flow to the kidneys and an increase in the rate at which the kidneys filter the blood. As a result you need to urinate more often. Your bladder may be squashed in the last trimester, making the urge to urinate very uncomfortable and even more frequent. This may increase the risk of bladder infections.

The kidneys are less efficient at absorbing filtered glucose, so glucose might appear in your urine, even in non-diabetic mothers.

You feel and look different

While many of the changes of pregnancy are miraculous ways in which your body nurtures your baby, some changes are more about your appearance.

POSTURE CHANGES

Your posture will change during pregnancy. As your baby grows, your centre of gravity changes and you will lean backwards to compensate for this. Your tummy muscles are less able to contract and keep the lower back in proper alignment, so the usual curves in your upper spine straighten out, and the curve in the lumbar spine increases. This predisposes you to backache.

The ligaments and joints of the pelvis soften and loosen, increasing the mobility of the joints in the pelvis, and providing more space for the baby to pass through at birth. This can cause pain and tenderness, as well as instability, leading to the waddling gait of pregnancy. The increased movement of the joints can also result in entrapment of nerves, for example the sciatic nerve, causing pain and sometimes numbness or pins and needles in the buttocks and legs – so-called sciatica.

PREGNANCY GLOW

Some changes occurring in pregnancy will alter your appearance:

- **Skin** – You may experience various skin changes, including all or some of the following:
  » Your blood vessels dilate and deliver more blood flow to your skin, leaving you glowing or possibly causing spider veins to develop under the skin.
  » The hormones of pregnancy increase pigmentation, so that existing pigmented spots darken and new pigmented patches appear. Pigmentation of the face usually affects the forehead, nose and cheeks and is called melasma or chloasma.
  » The nipples and areolea (area around the nipples) darken, and your belly button may also be affected.
  » The *linea nigra* – a dark line running down the middle of your abdomen – appears later in pregnancy.
  » The rapid stretching of skin can result in stretch marks. These affect the abdomen, thighs, buttocks, upper arms and breasts.
  » Itching is common in pregnancy.
  » Little skin tags often form where there is friction – under your breasts or in the armpits.

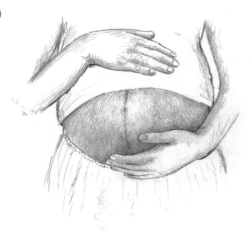

- **Hands** – Increased blood flow to your palms may cause a red appearance, called *palmar erythema*, and you may have sweaty palms as the activity of the sweat and sebaceous glands also increases.
- **Feet** – Swelling of the feet is common in pregnancy, particularly towards the end. Your feet may actually increase temporarily by half a shoe size or more owing to the stretching of the ligaments that hold the feet bones in place, resulting in their spreading.
- **Hair** – Both your hair and nails grow faster in pregnancy. You may notice an increase in fine, downy body hair, and there is usually an increase in pigmented hair, especially pubic hair, which can become quite long and might grow upwards onto the lower abdomen.
- **Face** – Your face often becomes fuller and rounder as pregnancy progresses.
- **Teeth** – Your gums may become more prone to infection and bleeding.

Nasty niggles

While pregnancy symptoms are largely signs of the miracle of your body's changes to nurture a growing baby, there are a few niggles that are more irritating than positive.

A LEAKY BLADDER

Incontinence, or leakage of urine, might occur in pregnancy – usually toward the end. It often occurs when you laugh or sneeze (stress incontinence), or when you just don't get to the loo in time (urge incontinence). This is due to the temporary changes of pregnancy. Wear a pad, if necessary, and do Kegel exercises (see p. 109).

> **Making sense**
>
> **Kegel exercises** tighten the muscles that hold your pelvic organs (bladder, rectum and the uterus) in place. These muscles are activated when you try to cut off urine midstream.

SNORING

You will possibly snore due to increased blood flow and congestion of the nasal passages.

FLATULENCE

You may burp and fart more, thanks to the sluggishness of your digestive tract.

HEARTBURN

As the sphincter at the entrance to the stomach relaxes, it allows the acid contents of the stomach to rise into the oesophagus, causing heartburn and reflux.

MORNING SICKNESS

This is a misnomer as nausea and vomiting can occur all day. Some say the purpose is to protect you from taking in noxious or toxic food. Any mom who went off mangoes or bananas may question the truth of that. It does, however, peak at a time when your foetus is the most vulnerable – before 12 weeks – so there may be some truth in this theory.

FATIGUE

You will be tired, especially in the first trimester. Like morning sickness, the fatigue you feel may be protective, preventing you from over-exerting yourself.

Some days these body changes will feel awesome and the next you may have a bad day — not loving your swollen feet and achy back. Remember in those moments that your body is going through huge, miraculous changes. Go with it. Enjoy your changing shape, recognise that almost all changes are for a reason and are temporary, and focus on the positive.

YOUR DIET

Sindi knows that her diet and what she consumes during pregnancy have a direct bearing on her baby's development both in the womb and throughout life. In her first trimester she barely gained more than a kilogram owing to severe morning sickness but now she is tempted by anything sweet and feels constantly hungry. The worst part is that she can't face anything healthy and has developed a craving for fatty chips, burgers and bread. With all this unhealthy eating, it's not surprising that she has put on 9 kg already, adding the anxiety of how she would get rid of any excess weight.

You know the significance of pregnancy or you would not be reading this. You also know that it's a once-off opportunity for this child — you don't get to go back and do it over. It's nine months of your life but will have far-reaching effects, so do it properly:

- You get the opportunity to provide the building blocks for every cell for your child's entire life — eat consciously, making each mouthful count.
- How much weight you gain will be what you need to lose afterwards — eat healthily, with that in mind.
- New research is showing that the quality of your diet in pregnancy has far-reaching consequences for your baby, impacting on the risk of cancer, cardiovascular disease, hypertension and diabetes throughout life.

SAFE AND UNSAFE BEAUTY TREATMENTS

There will be days in pregnancy when you need a lift. You will hear conflicting opinions regarding beauty treatments, but these are our recommendations:

Hair colouring – You may be concerned about exposure to chemicals used in hair dye and highlights. The reality is that the risk only exists when levels are exceptionally high, which is not the case when colouring hair. It is therefore safe to dye your hair in pregnancy. Wear gloves and be in a well-ventilated room. If you are worried, use henna rather than dye.

Highlighting is safe as chemicals come into contact with the hair and not the scalp.

Skin treatments
- Treatments high in Vitamin A and its derivatives (e.g. Differin gel, Retin-A) should not be used in pregnancy.
- Botox and fillers should be avoided in pregnancy.
- Topical erythromycin (Zineryt) for acne is safe in pregnancy.

Hair removal – Your skin is often more sensitive in pregnancy and you might find hair removal a little more painful than usual.
- Waxing, shaving and plucking are all safe.
- Laser and electrolysis should be avoided.

Massage – A relaxing massage is a good idea and is safe.
- From halfway through pregnancy, avoid lying flat on your back.
- Aromatherapy using diluted essential oils may be beneficial, but should only be used with advice from a therapist who understands the safety of oils in pregnancy. Some aromatherapy oils are toxic in the first trimester and others may trigger uterine contractions.
- Similarly, certain reflexology points are said to stimulate the uterus. As long as these areas are avoided, reflexology is fine.

Facials, manicures and pedicures are safe.

Tanning – Do not use tanning beds in pregnancy.

- There are substances that *your* body can process but that have a negative effect on your baby – like alcohol and certain medications. You need to eat and drink with your developing foetus in mind.
- Problematic diet in pregnancy can contribute to pregnancy complications, such as gestational diabetes. This can be very problematic for your baby – causing complicated labour, birth defects, prem labour and long-term changes in your baby's metabolism.

The media is full of conflicting advice on diet in pregnancy. You know that alcohol has risks but may be told that a drink a day is fine. You love your low-carb eating plan but have heard that ketones are bad for babies and thus a low-carb diet is irresponsible. You know that your baby needs omega 3 for brain growth but are warned against eating fish. The contradictions go on and on. Let's debunk a few of these myths.

Carbs versus fats

After the Second World War, most dietary advice promoted a diet made up of the five food groups, with low-fat foods and a predominance of carbohydrates in meals. In recent years, diets such as Banting and Paleo have been advocating a move towards low carbs and higher fats.

Pregnancy is not the time to try new diets. If you are on a Banting or Paleo diet and this method of eating has worked well for you, there is no reason that you cannot continue. Likewise, if you are doing well on a food groups diet, there is no need to change the way you eat.

IS IT SAFE TO FOLLOW A LOW-CARB DIET DURING PREGNANCY?

The controversy over the safety of a low-carb diet in pregnancy stems from contradictory opinions on what constitutes a low-carb diet, and misconceptions about ketosis (using fat for energy).

What is low carb? For the purpose of this book, low carb does **not** mean avoiding fruits and starchy vegetables. It does mean limiting processed grains and sugars. A balanced diet for pregnancy should include all fresh seasonal fruit and vegetables, hormone-free dairy products, natural whole grains and all fats and proteins. If you have a medical condition that is associated with blood sugar issues, such as gestational diabetes or preeclampsia, or you simply want to prevent excess weight gain, you may rest assured that it is safe to eat a low-carb diet as defined above.

Traditionally most pregnancy diets recommended that a woman eat an arbitrary minimum of 175 g of carbs per day. Research now shows that it is safe to eat less than this. The source of the carbs is more important than the total carb volume. Even on a seemingly low-carb diet, you will most likely consume about 100 g of naturally occurring carbs in nuts, seeds, fruit, vegetables, dairy and legumes. If you want to reduce your carb intake, cut out refined grains, junk food and added sugar. This will leave more room for nutrient-dense foods that provide a growing baby with essential nourishment.

Understanding ketosis. It is widely but incorrectly accepted that nutritional ketosis during pregnancy is harmful to a developing foetus. When carb levels are inadequate, protein and free fatty acids are used to produce glucose (a simple carbohydrate) in a process called nutritional ketosis. Nutritional ketones are the by-product and provide about a third of the developing baby's brain energy.

So, in a nutshell, a low-carb diet is safe, but it is important to acknowledge that, in addition to nutritional ketones, your growing foetus requires glucose for energy and growth. The important thing is that you consume enough calories to maintain normal blood sugar levels so that your baby will get just the right mix.

Gestational diabetes (too much sugar in the blood) affects one in five pregnancies and places you and your baby at significant health and developmental risk. It is considered a very serious condition in pregnancy and your caregiver will monitor the sugar in your urine at each visit.

High-carbohydrate diets, particularly those with sugary foods, lots of fruit juice and processed carbs (flour, bakes and cookies), cause your body to release insulin to stabilise your blood sugar. Like many organs, your pancreas is under pressure in pregnancy and may not be able to secrete enough insulin to cope with sugars you ingest.

Eating too many simple carbohydrates will exacerbate this. Such a diet, in combination with producing inadequate insulin, creates the perfect storm for gestational diabetes. Gestational diabetics should be referred to a dietician, but the basics of dietary management are to:

- avoid sugar and refined grain-based foods (bread and cookies) entirely;
- always eat healthy carbs (vegetables, dairy and fruit) in combination with fats or proteins (nut-butter, fish, nuts, hemp seed, eggs, chicken and steak) to stabilise your blood sugar; and
- not drink your carbs – no fruit juice or sugary sodas.

For a more in-depth study of using a low-carb diet to manage gestational diabetes, it is worth having a look at http://realfoodforgd.com/.

Allergenic foods for infants

With increased allergies in children, it became common to recommend that pregnant moms avoid allergenic foods such as nuts and even fish in pregnancy in an attempt to prevent them. What resulted was the opposite – an increase in the allergy epidemic among populations who followed this advice, while those who have always eaten diets rich in nuts and fish retained a lower allergy profile. Recent research shows that your eating allergenic foods (as long as you are not allergic to them yourself) may actually protect your baby from developing food allergies later.

Alcohol in pregnancy

Alcohol is a teratogen, which means it is toxic to the developing brain – it affects the formation and migration of brain cells.

Alcohol abuse leads to foetal alcohol syndrome (FAS), which involves mental retardation among other severe abnormalities. Moderate alcohol use can lead to foetal alcohol effects (FAE) with mild learning problems and ADHD and other conduct disorders as a consequence. The problem is that we simply do not know how much is too much.

It is believed that some babies' brains have the resilience to cope with a degree of alcohol without negative consequences, while others' brains are vulnerable and a small amount of alcohol or one binge-drinking session at the wrong time in pregnancy will have devastating consequences. The truth is that you don't know your baby's resilience to this teratogen and so the most sensible advice is to abstain altogether for the first trimester when brain cell migration is at its peak.

For the rest of pregnancy one or two small drinks up to twice a week is the most you should consume. A small drink is a single measure of spirits, 218 ml bear or 76 ml wine.

HEALTHY EATING FOR PREGNANCY

Since everything you eat passes from your digestive system, into your bloodstream, through the placenta and to your new baby, there are five points to consider when you listen to advice on diet in pregnancy:

1. Your diet needs to provide all the **nutrients** (building blocks) for all your baby's growing needs, and specific **micronutrients** ensure his brain and organ development is on track to meet his genetic potential.
2. Your nutrition needs to sustain an entire new organ – the placenta – and sustain your **energy levels** to nurture this organ, your own body and your growing foetus.
3. You need to be conscious of your **weight gain**. Gain too little and your baby may have stunted growth. Gain too much and there can be health consequences for you and your baby, and you may battle to lose it after your baby's birth.
4. In pregnancy, you are at risk for certain conditions related to diet – specifically **gestational diabetes**. Your diet has a direct effect on this.
5. **Fluids, and water specifically,** are essential for all body functions and, since much of your weight gain in pregnancy is water (more blood, amniotic fluid and fluid retention in preparation for birth), you obviously need to keep well hydrated in pregnancy.

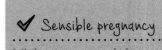 **Sensible pregnancy**

While it is not a good idea to eat for two, you will do well to eat with two in mind – not two adults, but two individuals with very specific needs.

Macronutrients

The main components of food are macronutrients – fats, protein and carbohydrates. These nutrients are found in all healthy food sources, including nuts and seeds, fruit, vegetables, meat and legumes, and are digested and processed to provide micronutrients (vitamins and minerals) and energy. This energy in turn is the basis for all essential body functions. During pregnancy, both you and your baby need micronutrients and energy. For this reason, the amount of macronutrients you need increases when you are pregnant.

The following nutrients are essential:

PROTEIN TO PROMOTE GROWTH

Protein is crucial for your baby's growth. In the first trimester, protein intake helps stabilise your blood sugar and helps with early-morning nausea. During the second and third trimesters, your protein intake supports your baby's growth and keeps your muscles strong. Most women need an extra 80 g of protein each day. Some research shows that adequate protein lowers the risk of complications such as preeclampsia.

Eat this: You should include two portions of protein (a palm size is one portion) with each meal and one protein portion with each snack to ensure adequate protein intake. Lean meat, poultry, fish and eggs are great sources of protein. Other options include dried beans and peas, tofu, dairy products and peanut butter.

CARBOHYDRATES FOR ENERGY

Healthy, unprocessed, naturally occurring carbohydrates have an important role to play in our diet as they contain micronutrients, fibre and water.

Eat this: Foods that fall into this group are seasonal fruits and all vegetables, legumes and nuts. You should have three to four fruit portions per day during pregnancy, eaten whole with skin where appropriate, and preferably raw and seasonal fruits only. All colours and types of vegetable should be eaten regularly. These include orange and yellow vegetables such as sweet potato, butternut and gem squash. Vegetables should be steamed, rather than boiled, or eaten raw where possible.

Avoid this: Fruit juices, dried fruit and fruit sugar.

FATS FOR ENERGY
Healthy fats provide double the amount of calories for half the volume of food compared with any other nutrient. This is helpful, especially when your stomach capacity decreases in the third trimester. Fats also contain essential fatty acids (omega 3), which are critical for the organ and brain development of the growing baby, as well as for building your and your baby's immune systems.

Eat this: You should focus on healthy sources of fat like cooked fish, meat (including red meat), butter, eggs, olive oil, coconut oil, avocado, tree nuts, seeds and dairy.

Micronutrients
These are needed in tiny quantities to maintain your and your baby's health. They include vitamins and minerals. Foods that contain a high ratio of micronutrients are said to be nutrient dense as there is more goodness than empty calories in the food. These are the types of food you should eat when you are pregnant.

FOLATE AND FOLIC ACID TO PREVENT BIRTH DEFECTS
Folate is a B vitamin that helps prevent serious abnormalities of the brain and spinal cord, such as *spina bifida*. Lack of folate in a pregnancy diet may also increase the risk of preterm delivery. The synthetic form of folate in supplements and fortified foods is known as folic acid. Supplementing with 400 μg folic acid per day, in combination with a healthy diet before conception and during pregnancy, is important.

Eat this: Fortified cereals contain folate. Leafy green vegetables, citrus fruits and dried beans and peas are good sources of folate.

CALCIUM TO STRENGTHEN BONES
You and your baby need calcium for strong bones and teeth. Calcium also helps your circulatory, muscular and nervous systems run normally. If there's not enough calcium in your pregnancy diet, the calcium your baby needs will be leached from your bones. While calcium requirements in pregnancy increase, absorption of calcium also increases, so routine supplementation is not necessary. If you are concerned that your diet does not cover your needs, daily supplementation of 500 mg of calcium is adequate.

Sometimes a calcium supplement, **with** vitamin D, of 1 g daily is specifically recommended from 12 weeks onward for women at increased risk of preeclampsia, as it might reduce the risk.

Eat this: Dairy products are the richest sources of calcium. If you are lactose intolerant, soy and almond milk are excellent sources. Leafy greens, seafood such as sardines and salmon, legumes, tofu and molasses are also good sources.

IRON TO PREVENT ANAEMIA
Your body uses iron to make haemoglobin, the part of the red blood cells that carries oxygen to your tissues. During pregnancy your blood volume increases to accommodate changes in your body and to help

your baby make his entire blood supply. As a result, your iron requirement nearly doubles to 27 mg per day. If you don't get enough iron, you may become fatigued and more susceptible to infections. The risk of preterm delivery and low birth weight may also increase.

Eat this: Red meat, poultry and fish are good sources of iron. Other options include green leafy vegetables and tree nuts. Eating foods rich in vitamin C can help with iron absorption.

OMEGA 3 FOR THE BRAIN AND EYES

The omega 3 fatty acid, DHA, is found in high concentrations in the brain, eyes and central nervous system. Links have been made between a diet rich in fish during pregnancy and smarter babies. It is important to eat foods high in omega 3 specifically during the second and third trimesters of pregnancy, which is a time for important brain development.

You may be advised to discontinue omega supplements from 37 weeks as there is a theory that they may increase bleeding.

Eat this: Foods high in these essential fats include fatty fish like salmon, tuna and pilchards. Nuts and seeds like flaxseed are also high in these special fats.

> ### Making sense
> . . . .
> **Pica**
> If you find you are craving very strange things, you may be suffering from Pica. Pica is the term given to cravings for non-nutritive substances. These can include ice, ash, chalk and paper. Pica sometimes occurs because of a deficiency of certain nutrients (see p. 80).

Fluids

Your body needs more water in pregnancy. Your blood volume increases and your body is replacing amniotic fluid each day. Being hydrated helps with constipation, prevents urinary tract infections, reduces swelling and can relieve headaches.

Adequate fluid intake, including water in food, is 3 ℓ per day of which approximately 8–10 cups should be water and beverages. Water intake does depend on climate and exercise. Sensible advice is that your urine should be pale yellow or clear. If you feel thirsty you are not drinking enough.

Avoid gassy or caffeine-filled cold drinks, and check that the water you drink is safe.

Supplements

The amount of nutrients available to your baby is entirely dependent on your nutritional status. If you are eating a well-balanced diet of fresh food, your baby will receive most of the nutrients he needs. For this reason it is essential for you to maintain a good and healthy lifestyle during pregnancy. However, even with the best diet, there are certain key micronutrients that you will need to supplement.

Must have	If inadequate diet
• Folic acid 400 μg • Vitamin D 10 μg	• Calcium 500 mg • Iron 27 mg • Omega 3

Most of the transfer of vitamins and minerals occurs in the last trimester (after 28 weeks of pregnancy). Premature babies therefore lose out on this and require additional vitamins and minerals, which are given to premature babies from 7 to 10 days of life.

Weight gain

There is no one-size-fits-all approach to pregnancy weight gain. How much weight you need to gain depends on various factors, including your pre-pregnancy weight and body mass index (BMI).

To calculate BMI, divide your weight (kg) by your height (m), then divide the answer again by your height (m). Consider these general guidelines for pregnancy weight gain:

- If you are overweight before you fall pregnant (BMI over 25) you should gain 7–11 kg.
- If you are normal weight, you can gain 11–16 kg.
- If you are underweight, with a BMI under 18,5, you need to put on closer to 12–18 kg.
- If you are carrying twins or multiples, you will gain more weight.

Excessive weight gained will be difficult to lose and increases your risk for gestational diabetes. If you gain more than the recommended amount during pregnancy and you don't lose the weight after your baby is born, the excess kilograms carry life-long health risks. It's important to avoid overeating and to make healthy choices.

Although pregnancy isn't the time to lose weight, if you are overweight to start with, it's important to limit your weight gain as follows:

- Eliminate all refined carbohydrates and grains from your diet.
- Include vegetables and salads with all meals.
- Eat fresh (not dried) fruit up to a maximum of two to three portions per day.
- Have salads and vegetables with proteins such as a chicken breast rather than a fast food take-away.
- Eat sliced fruit or yoghurt instead of a biscuit or sugary treat.
- Include nuts and seeds daily.

HEALTHY PREGNANCY DIET

The increased requirements of pregnancy can be met by increasing your dietary intake by 300 calories per day. A healthy pregnancy diet should include:

Food type	Portions per day	Portion size	Foods
Leafy veggies	>3 portions	1 cup	Spinach, broccoli, cauliflower, salad greens and many others
Starchy veggies	2–3 portions	½ cup ready to eat	Butternut, sweet potato and gem squash

Food type	Portions per day	Portion size	Foods
Fruit	3–4 portions	I medium fruit, ¼ melon slice, 12 grapes, 2 strawberries, ¾ cup blueberries, raspberries, mixed berries	Apples, citrus, pears, berries, melon, grapes, stone fruit
Protein	8–12 portions	I egg	Omega-3 enriched or free-range eggs are best
		I palm-sized portion of meat or chicken	Beef, lamb, pork, chicken and others; grass-fed is best
		At least 2–3 palm-sized portions of fish per week	Low mercury fish – salmon, trout, tuna, snoek, sardines, herring, haddock, shrimp and many others; wild-caught fish is best
Dairy	2–4 portions	I cup	Buttermilk, full cream yoghurt and milk
		I matchbox size piece	Cheese
Legumes	I–2 portions	½ cup	Cooked legumes, peanuts, peas, beans, lentils, carob and soya
Fat	4–8 portions	¼ cup nuts, seeds	Almonds, walnuts, sunflower seeds
		I tsp fats and oils	Coconut oil, butter, lard, olive oil and cod liver oil
Grains	I portion	½ cup cooked grains	Quinoa, millet, spelt, oats, rice

NOTE: Fruit, legumes and starchy veggies can be interchanged.

EXERCISE

There are enormous benefits to exercising during pregnancy. Exercise will help you feel good, improve your posture and limit some pregnancy niggles like backache, swelling and fatigue. In addition, exercise may help prevent gestational diabetes. It is beneficial to be fit for labour, birth and motherhood, so it's worth making sure you prepare in pregnancy.

If you have always been pretty fit and active, you can continue with your exercise regime. Make sure you work out within your comfort limits and go for low-impact sports. Your sense of balance will change so sports that require balance, like cycling, horse riding and trail running, may become tricky for you and endanger your baby if you fall.

If you are a competitive athlete, seek advice from your caregiver, who will recommend what is safe for you and your baby.

If you are a bit of a couch potato and have not exercised before, it is really worth starting to exercise now. A good idea is to walk three times a week and do a yoga or Pilates class weekly too.

> ✔ Sensible pregnancy
>
> **Exercise intensity**
> While exercising during pregnancy is good for you, you should limit your intensity to around 60% of your usual maximum intensity.

RECOMMENDED EXERCISE FOR PREGNANCY

- Brisk walking
- Yoga
- Stationary cycling
- Pilates
- Swimming
- Step machines

- Tennis is generally safe but changes in balance during pregnancy may affect rapid movements.
- Running is fine in moderation, especially if you were doing so regularly before your pregnancy.

PROCEED WITH CAUTION

Like diet, exercise is best done in moderation. In addition, you need to consider these heightened risks in pregnancy:

- **Lying on your back** – From the second trimester onwards, as your baby gets bigger, you may find you become breathless when you lie on your back. This happens because the uterus presses down on the vein that returns blood to the heart. When doing exercises such as yoga or Pilates rather lie on your side.

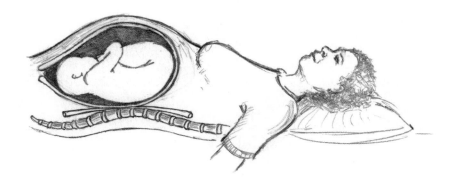

- **Overheating** – Overheating caused by sitting in a sauna or steam room is bad for the foetus, as your core temperature is already raised. Exercising per se is not likely to significantly alter your temperature but exercising on a very hot day or in a closed or heated room – such as heated yoga – is not advisable.
- **Falls** – Your sense of balance will be affected by having a new centre of gravity and you do want to avoid the risk of falls and injury.
- **Injury** – Your ligaments are all more lax than before pregnancy owing to the pregnancy hormone relaxin. This means that you are at risk for ankle sprains and ligament strains. Be aware of this by avoiding running on irregular surfaces (trail running) and avoid overstretching.
- **Exercises to be avoided** include trail running, rowing machines, power plates, heavy weight lifting, cycling and sit ups from 30 weeks on, contact sport such as judo or karate, snow- or water-skiing or -boarding, kite-surfing, scuba diving.
- **Stop exercising if you experience unusual**
    - » nausea;
    - » shortness of breath;
    - » bleeding or leakage of fluid;
    - » increased contractions;
    - » dizziness;
    - » fainting;
    - » pain.

The esSense of your changing body

- Pregnancy is the ultimate miracle of life. Your body changes to nourish a foreign being. You build a new organ, the placenta, for this purpose and each system within your body – circulatory, respiration, waste and digestion – caters for this new life.

- In addition to weight gain, your appearance will change more subtly in terms of posture, skin, hair and face.

- During pregnancy you may experience the inconvenience of a leaky bladder, snoring, heartburn, morning sickness and fatigue.

- You need to eat a balanced diet with limited sugar and processed carbohydrates in order to maintain healthy growth of your baby and reasonable weight gain.

- You will gain between 7 and 18 kg depending on your pre-pregnancy weight. Only 3–3,5 kg of this is baby and the rest is made up of blood, water, uterine muscle and fat.

- Supplements cover nutritional bases that may not be adequately taken in via your diet, such as folic acid, calcium, iron and omega 3.

- Exercise in moderation will elevate your mood, maintain healthy weight gain and keep you fit for labour and birth.

CHAPTER 3

It takes a village to raise a child

Julie's first pregnancy in her early twenties was very stressful. A young mom in an unstable marriage, was also working hard in a challenging job. After Mia's birth, she had no support. Looking back, she knows she was depressed and anxious throughout that pregnancy and her little one's early years were marked with marital tension, fights and eventually divorce. Although she swore never to remarry, when she fell in love with Jake, having his baby was the most natural route to go. This entire pregnancy had been different. Julie feels emotionally stable, she is supported in a loving relationship and her days are full of delight, knowing that this little one is her bonus baby. But she knows that this nine-month period will bring about dramatic changes to her relationship with Jake, her first-born and their respective extended families.

Whether this is your first or a subsequent pregnancy, always be aware of your emotions and those of the people around you. Pregnancy is an emotionally turbulent time, not just because of your hormones but also because of the dramatic shift in your life – one that you will start to notice more and more as your pregnancy progresses.

During the nine months of pregnancy, you are not only growing a baby – you are growing a mother too. You will develop a picture of the baby you will have, of the parent your partner will be and of a 'fantasy mother' – you. The way in which your *fantasy* matches your experience after birth may influence your mood and emotions in the early days.

> **TASKS OF PREGNANCY AND EARLY MOTHERHOOD**
>
> There are four tasks of pregnancy and early motherhood:
> - Physically caring for your baby
> - Emotionally nurturing your baby
> - Adjusting to motherhood
> - Creating a support system for you and your baby

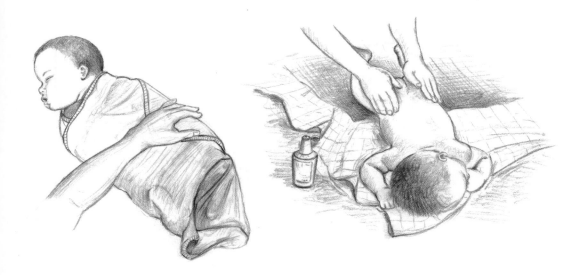

EMOTIONAL LIFE OF MOM

When Julie looks back, she can identify emotional issues that she had battled with in her earlier pregnancy – she had not really felt ready to have a baby and the thought of being the one to manage work and the responsibility of a baby felt like an unfair sacrifice. Even seeing her friends drink a glass of wine when she had to abstain made her resent those around her and, if she was honest, at times she resented her unborn baby. She was in no way ready to take on the daunting and life-changing role she had been thrust into. People spoke of postnatal depression but Julie felt as low during pregnancy as she did for the next few years. She now knows antenatal depression is as common as postnatal, and may precede low moods and anxiety after birth.

Your emotions leading up to the birth of your baby are affected by both pregnancy hormones and the life stage shift.

If you are having a second baby, you may worry about how you can share your love and how a new sibling will affect your first-born. There will be days when you feel scared and others when you are excited.

Women respond differently to the change of role and the hormones of pregnancy. You may, like many women, glow and love the preggy phase, embracing the dream of being a mom. On the other hand, you may feel scared and low. Your body may feel foreign and not your own. You may even feel slightly conflicted by the idea of a human life growing within you. If you are battling, remember that you are not alone. Talk to someone you trust or seek professional help.

Emotions in pregnancy

No two pregnancies are the same and your emotions will be influenced by many factors, including your age and whether this is a planned or 'surprise' pregnancy. That said, there are phases you will probably move through that are fairly common.

FIRST TRIMESTER

During the first 13 weeks of pregnancy, your attention will be on the physical changes in your body occurring almost daily. One day you feel fine and the next your breasts are sore; a day later your sense of smell heightens and a week later your tummy feels bloated. Your emotions will be affected by these physical changes — when you are tired, sore or ill, you may feel low and anxious.

Another common feeling in the first trimester is the fear of losing your baby. It is estimated that 15 per cent of pregnancies end in miscarriage, sometimes before a woman even knows she is

---

FEELING DOWN IN PREGNANCY

You know you should be elated – you have been blessed with a new life. But you just don't really feel that great. It may be that you are very anxious or you may actually be depressed at the thought of having a baby. This is known as *antenatal distress* and is more common than many think. It may come and go throughout pregnancy.

How to cope

If you are anxious, irritable or quite low before the birth of your baby, try to get plenty of sleep, rest and exercise, and eat well. Your emotions are linked to your *physical state* too.

If you have a history of depression or anxiety and have stopped taking your *medication*, you may need to start again. There are many options that are considered safe for your baby – it is essential that you discuss this with your doctor.

Although antenatal distress does not mean that you will automatically experience *postnatal depression*, research has shown that there is a link, so speak to your caregiver about these feelings.

Remember that it takes a village to raise a child and this starts in pregnancy. Ask for help, speak to friends or contact PNDSA (Post Natal Depression Support Association). They will help you prepare emotionally for the journey. (See http://www.pndsa.org.za/.)

---

pregnant. The fear for your child's safety will not leave you for the rest of your life. However, the magic 13-week milestone does settle most moms' minds, as the risk of pregnancy loss is substantially reduced after the first trimester.

Hormonal changes and the developing placenta take a toll on your energy levels and may leave you tired and feeling sick. These physical symptoms may reduce your resilience and sense of wellbeing, and result in extreme mood swings – one minute you are laughing and the next crying. You may feel like you don't know yourself.

SECOND TRIMESTER

The second trimester brings with it the glow of pregnancy – not only do the difficult symptoms of early pregnancy (fatigue, nausea and bloating) dissipate, but you will start to feel a general sense of wellbeing and joy.

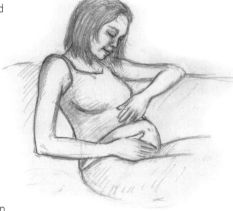

You may find this is the first time you start to bond with your baby – you have more peace of mind that the pregnancy is safe, you will probably see your baby on ultrasound, the dreaded early tests for foetal anomalies have passed and you start to feel your little one move.

During this trimester you may start to battle a bit with your changing body image – your clothes will become tight and you may feel fat – at a stage when you don't yet look pregnant but can't fit into your old jeans.

Some women, especially if they have been independent and in charge of their own career, may find a fear of dependence on their partner develops. This vulnerability can cause some friction in your relationship, as you feel a little less attractive and a whole lot more dependent than before. It is important to express these emotions and ask your partner to bear with your insecurities – they will pass as you embrace the new role in the months and years to come.

THIRD TRIMESTER

As the end approaches, your mind will become preoccupied with the birth and safe arrival of your baby. This can lead to anxiety as those late pregnancy niggles and pains become cause for concern.

You may fear the actual birth and wonder how you will cope with the pain. Becoming informed and attending an antenatal course is a wonderful way to sensibly manage pre-birth jitters.

Through the experience of pregnancy, you will grow as a person and you should be ready by the end to move into the new emotional phase of being a mom.

YOUR VILLAGE

The saying "It takes a village to raise a child" is true right from conception. You and your baby are not developing in a vacuum. You

---

Making sense

Tokophobia

A small percentage of women have a debilitating fear of childbirth – they avoid falling pregnant, or may have panic attacks at the thought of how the baby is going to be born. If you are preoccupied and paralysed with fear of birth, tell your doctor. Choosing a more predictable method of delivery, such as a planned epidural or Caesarean section, is often useful for moms who cannot face the thought of delivery.

are both being nurtured and affected by and affecting the world, society and your family who surround you – your village.

Dad

Most babies are born in the context of a relationship and this section takes that into account. If you are a same sex couple, please read the word 'mom' as primary carer and 'dad' as partner. If you are a single parent and do not have a partner to help share the load, you may feel that this section is not relevant. Try to find a support system within your village if that is the case.

Your partner will not be left unaffected by this pregnancy, and considering his role and emotions will protect your relationship. Your goals in this regard should be twofold:

- To protect your relationship, the stability of which will provide a secure base from which your child will explore the world.
- To nurture a close relationship between your baby and her dad.

PROTECT YOUR RELATIONSHIP

There will be times when Dad will have a tough time understanding your emotions, especially if you are tired and emotional. Try to give him a window on your world by expressing your feelings and anxieties with "I feel" messages, rather than "You …" statements. "I feel tired and need some help" rather than "You never help me".

Keep him feeling important. There will be a lot of attention on you and your baby but in years to come you will want to have protected your relationship, so make sure you keep a long-term view regarding his importance.

SEX IN PREGNANCY

Your sexual relationship is important in pregnancy and after. But it will be different. You may feel 'unsexy' and more functional than pretty but it may be that your partner actually still feels the desire to connect physically. Ask him how he sees you and whether he is interested in physical contact.

- If he is not interested, do not take it personally – he may fear hurting your baby through intercourse.
- If he is interested and you are not, try to find ways to satisfy his needs without intercourse per se. Or explain to him that you do not feel turned on.

Sex in pregnancy is different for everyone. For some, pregnancy enhances their sex life:

- You may feel more sexy and your partner may find your bump sensual.
- There is the freedom of sex without contraception, allowing more relaxed sex with greater tactile pleasure without a condom.
- Many women find themselves more aroused as pregnancy progresses because there is more blood in the breast and pelvic area.
- You may find the creativity of new positions a great turn-on.
- Many women experience more intense orgasms.

On the other hand, you may find pregnancy is a passion killer:

- Some women have reduced sex drive and battle to have an orgasm.

> ✔ Sensible pregnancy
> ....
> **Reasons to refrain from sex**
> - If you bleed after having sexual intercourse
> - If you are at risk of preterm labour
> - If your membranes have ruptured (waters have broken)
> - If you have a stitch around your cervix due to threat of a miscarriage
> - If your partner has an STD like herpes

- Either or both partners may battle to be intimate knowing there is a third person 'in the bed'. Imagining the baby so close to the area of penetration may be a turn-off.
- Many dads fear hurting the baby or may find they are not sexually attracted to their partner when she is pregnant.

Unless your caregiver says otherwise, sex in pregnancy is safe and does not risk harming your baby in any way. Try to keep a sense of humour and enjoy each other's bodies in this new phase.

Pregnancy may mean you need to try new positions:
- You kneel down or on all fours and your partner enters your vagina from behind.
- Lie side by side and your partner enters you from in front or behind.
- Your partner sits on a chair and you are on top of him facing forwards or backwards.

NURTURE YOUR BABY'S RELATIONSHIP WITH DAD

One of the greatest fears for many dads is the fear of not bonding with their baby. You get a head start on feeling your little one move and will connect more readily in the second trimester. Many dads worry that they will never feel the connection. To ensure he does connect, include him in the antenatal visits, in choosing names, nursery colour and birth method. Make sure he gets to feel your baby move whenever you can. Tell him how your baby will learn his voice too from the third trimester of pregnancy and encourage him to talk, read and sing to her.

On the day your baby is born, have Dad hold her skin to skin on his chest. This early touch releases oxytocin and has a wonderful impact on falling in love.

After the birth, include Dad in essential caregiving – nappy changes, bath time and burping. All daily activities hold the opportunity for bonding through touch.

Accept his offers of help and do not criticise the way he does the task. Rather praise or reinforce it – even if it's not the way you would have done it. This will empower Dad and invite further offers of help. Remember that not all dads are the same; some prefer being observers in the early days. This doesn't mean they love their baby any less. These dads will become more hands on when their baby is a little bigger and more fun.

Siblings

Julie is ready for her new baby to come. Her Caesarean section has been scheduled for tomorrow and this is her last evening as a mom of one. As she sits on Mia's bed and strokes the locks from her five-year-old's brow, she feels an overwhelming sense of sadness. Once the baby is born, Mia will no longer be her baby and she will have to share her mommy in the months to come. Julie wishes she could hold on to this moment for a while. Tomorrow it will all change.

As a second- or third-time mom, the night before you give birth will be one of the hardest in your parenting journey so far, as the realisation sets in that tomorrow your little baby is going to be a big sister. You will mourn the loss of her baby status as she graduates to older sibling.

This will never feel more real than when you see them together, big sister holding her tiny new sibling. She will seem

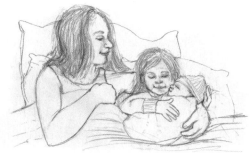

so big compared with the newborn. And knowing that her baby status is gone forever, even though she is only a little one herself, will pluck at your heartstrings.

There may be times after your new baby is born when you lose your cool and are irritable around your older children. You will be tired and your fuse may be short. You may be overcome with guilt, knowing that they did nothing wrong.

To ease the transition for older siblings you have to consider their emotional needs and help them find the words for their feelings. A special introduction to your new baby and creating windows of opportunity to connect with your other children is the best way to manage this.

TELLING YOUR CHILDREN YOU ARE PREGNANT

It is advisable to wait until you are into your second trimester, when the risk of losing the baby reduces substantially, before telling your child that you are pregnant. The best time to share the news will depend on your child's age and understanding. With a child under 18 months you may want to wait until you are showing.

With an older toddler or preschooler you should not wait too long after you have told others as there is a risk of someone slipping up and telling your little one before you get the chance. A good time to tell her is when you feel your baby move for the first time – around 20 weeks. This will make the concept of a life inside you a little more tangible.

Start laying the groundwork by pointing out pregnant friends and talk about the baby growing inside them. Then relate that to how she grew inside you before she was born. Once she has grasped that concept, simply tell her: "You are going to be a very special big sister because there is a baby growing in Mommy's tummy." Your older child or children need to be reassured that you will still be their mommy and they are still your 'babies'. The words you choose will depend on their age, but the principle remains the same.

INTRODUCING SIBLINGS TO THE NEW BABY

There are two trains of thought on taking siblings to the hospital. For most toddlers the excitement of going to see Mom and meet *their* new baby is a special event and their parents encourage this. Other parents feel that taking a toddler's germs into a maternity ward is not a good idea and prefer the older child to wait until Mom gets home. The decision will probably be based on how long you spend in hospital. If it is only overnight or you have your baby at home, your toddler will be able to meet his sibling and reunite with Mom quickly. A three- to four-day hospital stay is probably too long for a toddler to wait without seeing Mom and may exacerbate feelings of loss.

Get each child a gift – maybe a doll for the older sibling and a little teddy for the baby. Wrap these gifts and when your toddler meets her sibling for the first time, let them exchange gifts. Years later you will be amazed at how your older child recalls the gift her baby sibling gave her. Sitting on a bed or chair, let your older baby hold the new sibling, always being vigilant for your newborn's safety.

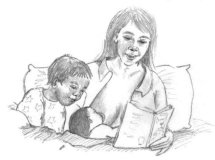

MANAGING BREAST-FEEDING

Many toddlers really battle with breast-feeding time because you are so incapacitated while your baby feeds – you can't get up or see to her needs during the feed. This is often when behavioural issues can arise. To avert this, put a pile of your toddler's favourite books on your feeding chair and call her to come and read. It will seem to her that the primary focus is the reading, not the feeding.

A 'ME-TIME' BOX

Both you and your toddler are likely to notice and feel sad about how little time you now have together. Try to set aside 10 minutes a day – maybe when your newborn is sleeping or when Dad gets home from work – to spend reconnecting.

Create a 'Me-time' box with six of your toddler's favourite toys. Include two of each toy – one for you and one for your toddler. Put away your phone and close the door so that you and your toddler have the room and time to yourselves.

Open the box and just focus on what your child plays with – if she chooses to play with the car, take a car out too and mimic what she does. Play at her pace and don't direct her play; just let her lead the way.

SHARING THE LOAD

An involved dad is essential for managing siblings after the birth of a new baby. Dad has to take over the care of the older sibling to a large degree, which has many benefits:

- A closer relationship with the older child and the feel-good effect of being needed and valuable
- Reduced risk of postnatal depression for Mom as she will not be as overwhelmed with the load of two or more children
- Less sibling rivalry and a closer relationship between the two siblings later

Other women

In many cultures the role of other women in nurturing a pregnant mother is regarded as very important. In the Western world it is not as prevalent, but one thing is certain – your relationship with other women will never be the same.

- You will see *your* mother in a new light. If your relationship is a good one, your mom will fill the role of nurturer and support. If you have a broken relationship, becoming a new mom may present an opportunity to mend ties.
- Differences between family norms can create tensions and anxiety. If women in your extended family tend to give unsolicited advice that you perceive as intrusive or critical, you will need to set boundaries before the birth of your baby.
- Distance yourself from people who increase your stress levels through unkind criticism. This is the root cause of toxic stress, which you must avoid at all cost. Create boundaries and ask your partner to help you manage difficult emotions.

Work

Your decision to work through your pregnancy and in the months after your baby's birth is a personal one, based on your job and what motivates you to work. For many this is not only a financial decision, but also

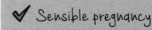 Sensible pregnancy

Practical ways to manage relationships
If you experience stressful and difficult emotions about friends, colleagues and family you need to manage these. Negative feelings are bad for you and your growing baby.

- Forgive the past and, if issues need to be addressed, do so.
- Choose to surround yourself with those who will contribute to your baby's life and be meaningful for your family unit, for example close family and friends in the same life stage as you.
- Don't try to control others' actions.
- Avoid toxic relationships – situations that create stress that you cannot control or shift.
- Find gratitude. Try to find something to be thankful for every day – it will raise your spirits.

part of their ambitions and need for stimulation. These are factors to consider if you are going to be a working mom.

Stress

When you are stressed, your body releases hormones to cope. This cortisol and adrenaline enter your blood stream and pass through the placenta to your baby. So your baby literally feels your stress. Stress per se is not necessarily a bad thing and experiencing low levels of stress can be beneficial for your baby's development. But prolonged periods of toxic stress may be harmful.

Toxic stress – stress we cannot escape or change and is long-lasting, such as inescapable conflict at work, physical or emotional abuse by a partner or colleague, or the illness and death of a parent – may negatively affect your child's emotional resilience in the long term. This type of ongoing stress creates pathways that are reinforced and can alter the wiring of your baby's brain.

In particular, the limbic system (the emotional seat of our brain) can become hyper-responsive to stressful events, resulting in lowered resilience through life.

Small stresses that are short-lived, such as a traffic jam or the normal work stress of deadlines, are transient. Although your baby feels the stress, it is unlikely to have a long-term negative effect.

Managing toxic stress

If you find yourself in a situation of extreme uncontrolled stress, try these strategies:

- Share the load with a trusted person. Disclosing your situation, no matter how stigmatised you may feel, will help you cope. Simply knowing that someone else knows about your problems can help you feel supported.
- Find non-judgemental support – someone you trust not to judge you but to listen and support you.
- Ask yourself: "What can I control?" If there is any way you can shift the pressure, do it. It may mean making changes to your job or career.

Breast-feeding and work life

Establishing breast-feeding is not an easy task and it takes time (more on this in Chapters 17 and 18). Having time and space is critical to establishing a good milk supply. Going back to work in the first four months might affect this so, if you have the choice not to work in the first four months after birth, it will benefit your breast-feeding.

Bonding

Connecting with your baby and her attachment to you are vital for all future relationships. This bond develops in the context of space, time and low pressure. It is precious time and passes in a flash. Taking time off from work and the pressures of life will give you space to bond with your baby.

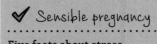

Sensible pregnancy

Five facts about stress and your baby

1. All stress you feel passes to your baby *in utero*.
2. Not all stress is bad for you or your baby.
3. Healthy stress and subsequent recovery can create resilience.
4. Toxic stress can be detrimental to your baby's brain wiring and long-term resilience.
5. Toxic stress is:
   - inescapable;
   - out of your control;
   - persistent;
   - usually interpersonal.

HINTS FOR THE OTHER HALF

Your ultimate role is as a containing vessel for the woman you love, as she nurtures and cares for your child. You become the buffer between the world and the mom–baby unit. Your partner will never be more vulnerable than in the first few months of motherhood. It's a tough time; there will be occasions when she is insecure and anxious. In this state of fear, it can be difficult to be the good mom she hoped to be; it may be hard for her to bond and meet her baby's emotional needs. This is where your role is vital. A partner should provide a safe space where Mom can care for and soothe and meet the basic needs of her baby without the pressures of the outside world.

Be involved:

- Where possible take two weeks' paternity leave.
- Be home for bath time and take over with the older sibling – bath time, story time and bedtime will be your special time and leave Mom free to focus on your newborn when she may be a little fractious.
- Assist with night feeds that fall before midnight. Let Mom stay in bed and take the baby to her for the feed, burp the baby and change the nappy between breasts, and after the feed, burp and swaddle her and settle her to sleep.
- Dad must sleep between midnight and 4 am. There is no point in having two sleep-deprived parents if Mom has to get up for the breast-feed anyway.
- For early morning feeds after 4 am, follow the same routine as for the feeds before midnight so Mom can rest and maybe doze while the baby feeds.
- If your baby is bottle-fed, share the night feeds on weekend nights to give Mom a good stretch of sleep.

The esSense of those around you in pregnancy

- The four tasks of motherhood start to develop in pregnancy – physically nurturing your baby, emotionally loving her, adjusting to being a mother and laying the groundwork for your baby's relationship with her family.

- In the first trimester your energy levels and your emotions will fluctuate a lot. Overall you will be largely focused on your changing body.

- Your second trimester is a period of energy and delight as you start to feel your baby move and your pregnancy is much more secure.

- As the pregnancy progresses, you may experience anxiety over the birth and your baby's safe delivery.

- Prioritise your relationship with your partner; this relationship is a vital base from which your baby will explore the world with confidence.

- Not all parents fall in love with their baby in pregnancy; bonding is a journey.

CHAPTER 4

Preparing for pregnancy

While they were enjoying sundowners on a Friday evening, Angela was astonished when Dave asked, "Shall we have a baby?" The question came out of nowhere. She thought that Dave wanted to focus on just the two of them and that having a baby was simply not on the agenda. A week after this surprise question, Angela has barely been able to think of anything else. Not only has she warmed to the idea, but she wants to embrace the journey and plan the route ahead. Many of her friends took time to fall pregnant and she realises that it may not happen immediately. Nonetheless, she wants theirs to be an informed decision.

The moment you decide to have a baby, you will begin to focus on falling pregnant and giving your baby the best possible start. This chapter will help you prepare your mind and body for conception.

CONCEPTION

Trying to fall pregnant is a loaded statement. It contains the sense of a goal, an expected outcome – that you may succeed or fail. It also entails an element of effort – the harder you try, the more likely a positive outcome. This creates unnecessary pressure.

Often this approach sets the tone for parenting – as something that is goal-directed and at which you can fail or be measured. It mirrors the future pressure of trying to be a good parent.

The truth is that, like parenting, conception, pregnancy and birth are a journey.

Stopping contraception

It is not necessary to wait for any prescribed period after stopping contraception before trying to conceive. Remember, though, that you may fall pregnant immediately, so don't stop contraception until you are ready for this.

The first bleed after you discontinue oral contraception is known as a withdrawal bleed. To ascertain when you conceived, so that you can calculate an accurate due date, it is helpful to wait until you've had your first natural menstrual period after the withdrawal bleed. However, this is not necessary for your baby's health. Should you conceive immediately, ultrasound scans are precise in dating pregnancy.

Best time to fall pregnant

There is no best time to fall pregnant. Since conception isn't always predictable and can take time, it is advisable to avoid rigid plans around timing, make sensible lifestyle changes and wait to see what happens.

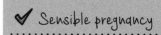

✔ Sensible pregnancy
. . . .

Fertility and contraceptives

Modern contraception is effective and you can conceive immediately after discontinuing the oral contraceptive pill, the contraceptive patch, the vaginal ring, the intrauterine device (IUD), the Mirena intrauterine system, the implant (Implanon) and barrier contraceptives (condoms, the diaphragm).

Although it is not always the case, return to fertility may be longer after discontinuing injectable contraceptives (Depo-Provera or Nur-Isterate).

You are fertile 48 hours before and 48 hours after ovulation and you ovulate 14 days before the start of your next menstrual period. The average menstrual cycle is 28 days; therefore ovulation occurs on day 14 (14th day from the start of the menstrual period) if you have a 28-day cycle. If you want to know more accurately, you need to track your cycle. It is quite normal for the cycle to vary by one or two days from one month to the next. Should you have a longer cycle, you will ovulate later than day 14. For example, for a 32-day cycle, ovulation occurs on day 18 (32 − 14 = 18).

KNOWING WHEN YOU ARE OVULATING

There is an enormous variation from one person to the next, and from one cycle to the next. Don't over-monitor your menstruation and ovulation, unless your cycle is irregular or you are battling to fall pregnant. In general, these are the signs you are ovulating:
• Your cervical fluid increases in volume and viscosity (like egg white).
• You may spot or experience pain on one side.

Home ovulation kits test for hormone levels in the urine. There are several user-friendly mobile phone apps available for tracking ovulation and fertile times (do a search on Google).

FALLING PREGNANT AFTER A PREVIOUS PREGNANCY
OR MISCARRIAGE

Ideally, wait a year before falling pregnant after a previous pregnancy. After a miscarriage or evacuation of uterus, you can try again after one normal period.

A healthy start

Having decided to stop contraception to fall pregnant, you will want to ensure that your baby has a healthy start. Other than diet, which was covered in Chapter 2, and managing stress (Chapter 3 p. 38), there are several important boxes to tick with regard to your health so that you don't worry about them once you are pregnant.

> ### Making sense
> . . . .
> **Evacuation of the uterus**, often incorrectly referred to as a 'D and C', refers to the procedure to remove the remains of the pregnancy from the cavity of the uterus, usually after a miscarriage.

INFECTIOUS DISEASES

Certain infections, if caught when you're pregnant, may cause abnormalities in your baby or put your pregnancy at risk. You may already be immune to these infections, either through vaccination or from a previous infection. Being vaccinated or having had the disease is not always a guarantee and you should have a simple blood test to confirm immunity.

If the blood test shows that you are not immune to these infections, you should consider vaccination against them and postpone falling pregnant until a month after receiving the vaccine. Discuss this with your GP, with particular reference to the following:

German measles (rubella) is a common viral infection. The symptoms are usually similar to that of mild flu, accompanied by a light rash. When a pregnant woman contracts German measles, her unborn foetus can become infected, resulting in Congenital Rubella Syndrome (CRS). The risk is highest in the first trimester (90 per cent), dropping considerably after 16 weeks. The effects on the pregnancy and foetus include miscarriage, intrauterine death, heart defects, cataracts and deafness, and many other malformations.

Chicken-pox (varicella) is a common viral infection. Again, it is usually a mild, flu-like illness characterised by an itchy rash that develops into small blisters. Pregnant women who become infected with chicken-pox have an increased risk of a severe infection, which may be complicated by pneumonia, hepatitis and encephalitis. If it is contracted before 28 weeks, there is a small risk that the foetus can become infected, resulting in Foetal Varicella Syndrome (FVS). This can produce eye and limb defects, and abnormalities of the brain and nervous system. The biggest risk to the foetus is if the mother has chicken-pox at the time of delivery when there is a 50 per cent chance of the newborn's catching varicella, with a significant risk of complications and death.

If you are exposed to chicken-pox or shingles during pregnancy and are not immune, you can ask for passive immunization with varicella zoster immuno globulin (VZIG), which is best given within 72 hours of exposure.

Influenza (flu) The 2009 swine flu pandemic is an example of how seasonal influenza can have serious complications for pregnant women, risking their lives and resulting in babies' being delivered prematurely. You *should* go for the seasonal flu vaccination as it is safe. Vaccination can be any time in winter, but it is best to have it done by April. If you are planning to fall pregnant, get vaccinated.

Pertussis, also known as whooping cough, can be a serious infection and babies are susceptible after delivery if a mother's antibody levels are insufficient. Although most babies are vaccinated against pertussis, immunity levels are declining in adults as a result of an adult booster not being given. Since immunity weakens over time, it is recommended that women planning pregnancy receive a booster against pertussis. In South Africa, the vaccine DTaP (Adacel) is not yet licensed for use during pregnancy and breast-feeding, so vaccination should be considered before pregnancy. This vaccine is registered for use in pregnancy abroad, and vaccination in the UK is recommended for all pregnant women after 28 weeks.

Genetic tests

There are no routine genetic tests that are recommended, unless there is a family history of conditions such as haemophilia or, in the case of Ashkenazi Jews, Tay-Sachs.

Sexually transmitted diseases (STDs)

Certain STDs can be transmitted to your unborn foetus. It is worthwhile knowing about these, as some can be treated, while others can be managed to reduce the risk of transmission to the foetus or the baby after birth. Women are usually tested once they are pregnant, although testing can be performed prior to pregnancy.

HIV infection is asymptomatic until the later stages of the disease. The risk of infecting the foetus if the mother is HIV positive can be reduced to almost zero with the use of antiretroviral medication during pregnancy.

The type of delivery and methods of feeding the baby may be influenced by the mother's HIV status.

Syphilis is asymptomatic for most of its course (the latent phase). It may result in intra-uterine death, premature birth and congenital abnormalities. Whilst it is rarely seen in developed countries, the incidence in South Africa as a whole is estimated at between 3 and 18 per cent. Syphilis can be treated with penicillin and the chance of congenital syphilis significantly reduced.

Hepatitis B is a viral infection causing acute infection (hepatitis), and chronic infection, leading to cirrhosis and liver failure. Chronically infected women are frequently asymptomatic, yet their babies may be infected at birth. Active and passive vaccination given at birth to such babies can prevent mother-to-child infection.

Herpes can be transmitted to your baby during childbirth. The risk exists even when there are no visible sores. In general, the risk of transmission is low, although infection of the newborn is very serious. If a woman catches a new (first) infection in the last six weeks of pregnancy, birth by Caesarean section is recommended.

TERATOGENS

A teratogen is an agent that can cause a birth defect (an abnormality in a foetus). You need to know about these to avoid them.

Medication Very few medications are known teratogens. Nevertheless, all medications used during pregnancy or while you are trying to fall pregnant should be checked with your doctor or pharmacist. Before stopping vital treatment you must discuss changing to different medication.

The following medication must be discontinued or replaced in consultation with your doctor before pregnancy:
- Certain anti-epileptic medication e.g. sodium valproate (Epilim)
- Acne treatments such as isotretinoin (Roaccutaine) and tetracycline
- Blood thinning or anti-clotting agents such as warfarin
- Lithium in the first trimester

Inform your doctor or caregiver if you have taken any of the above medications in pregnancy. In some cases, where the risks are low, medication such as anti-depressants might be continued once the risk–benefit ratio has been assessed.

Alcohol is the most common teratogen babies are exposed to, with potentially devastating consequences. A single binge-drinking episode may be harmful. It is recommended that pregnant women avoid alcohol altogether, especially in the first trimester. If you do drink, have no more than two standard units of alcohol up to twice a week *after* the first trimester. One standard unit is equivalent to 25 ml of spirits, 76 ml of wine or 218 ml beer.

Smoking is harmful to your unborn baby and increases the risks of many complications, including miscarriage, stillbirth, placenta issues resulting in low birth weight and prematurity. Smoking may also be associated with an increased risk of cleft palate or lip.

Cot death (sudden infant death syndrome or SIDS) and childhood asthma occur more frequently in babies born to smokers. There may also be a link between smoking and hyperactivity and attention disorders.

Consider pregnancy an excellent time to stop smoking; this is the most motivated you will ever be. It is beneficial to quit smoking at *any* stage during the pregnancy. Fortunately for some smokers, one of the effects of pregnancy is a dislike of cigarette smoke. Don't beat yourself up if you need help in the form of behavioural therapy or nicotine patches. Nicotine is a toxin, but nicotine replacement therapy (in the form of the patch, spray or gum) is better than smoking as exposure is then only to the nicotine and not the other toxins in cigarettes.

Second-hand smoke (exposure to the smoke of other cigarette smokers) is also detrimental.

Zika The World Health Organization has declared the Zika virus outbreak in South and Central America and the Caribbean a public health emergency of international concern. The infection, spread by mosquitoes, is not usually serious, but can result in microcephaly (a small head) and other brain abnormalities in babies of infected mothers.

Once you are pregnant, you should avoid travel to high-risk areas. Should travel be necessary the use of mosquito repellent and measures to prevent mosquito bites (wearing long-sleeved and -legged clothing, using mosquito nets) are recommended. If you have travelled to an affected area, inform your caregiver. If you have not had any symptoms, there is little reason for concern. If you are unwell, a blood test can detect the Zika virus. Ultrasound will usually show abnormalities that result from Zika virus infection.

Radiation In general, X-rays should be avoided. Having said that, the amount of radiation from one or two X-rays is unlikely to pose a risk to the foetus so, where indicated, X-rays can be performed but the foetus must be shielded as best as possible.

Heavy metals including lead and mercury should be avoided. The advice to increase intake of oily fish (to provide omega 3) is confusing when one reads that there might be high levels of mercury in oily fish. It is quite safe to eat up to three tins of tuna or two tuna steaks per week.

Caffeine does not cause abnormalities in the foetus, but there is research linking high caffeine intake to lower birth weight in babies. Recent guidelines recommend that daily caffeine intake should not exceed two cups of instant coffee or tea, and one mug of filter coffee. Remember that tea, cola or energy drinks, and chocolate also contain caffeine.

SUPPLEMENTS
Some supplements are important to ensure your baby gets the best chance for a healthy start.

Folic acid (folate) Scientific research indicates that you should take a folic acid supplement during the first 12 weeks of pregnancy, and ideally for a few weeks prior to pregnancy. Since folic acid levels are lower in women using oral contraceptive, you should start taking a folate supplement before you go off the pill.

Folate, a B group vitamin, is essential in the development of the foetus's brain and spinal cord (the neural tube). There is a significant reduction in the risk of your baby's having a cleft lip or palate or neural tube defects like *spina bifida* or anencephaly if you take folate supplements. The daily recommended supplement is 400 µg. Almost all multivitamins will contain this, and there are several preparations of folate alone. Many of these contain more than 400 µg and this is quite safe to take.

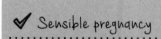

✔ Sensible pregnancy
. . . .

Toxic myths
When you are pregnant it is hard to separate myth from fact. Some of the things you may be told to avoid that are in fact most likely innocent include:
- Microwaves – unless the door of the microwave oven is damaged
- Aspartame
- Power lines
- Electric blankets
- MRI
- Ultrasound

New research suggests that a folic acid supplement prior to conception significantly reduces the risk of premature birth (possibly as much as 50 to 70 per cent), as well as the risk of low birth weight.

CHOOSING YOUR CAREGIVER

The single most important decision that directly affects your pregnancy and birth experience, is your choice of caregiver. This person becomes your partner, advising you, guiding you and collaborating with you to give you the pregnancy and birth experience you want – one that is safe for you and your baby. Before deciding on your caregiver, there are a number of important decisions to make.

Step 1: Your birth preference

Long before you fell pregnant, you probably had an idea about how you wanted to give birth and where. Most women do. Others remain undecided until near the end of their pregnancy. Essentially, there are two ways to deliver your baby.

- A natural – or vaginal – birth is so-called because it is birthing the way nature intended. Women have been giving birth vaginally from the beginning of time and we have not lost the ability to do so.
- A Caesarean birth, or C-section, is when your baby is delivered in a hospital via an incision in your abdomen. For centuries (the first written record goes back to the late 1500s), the C-section has been a life-saving safety net for a mother and baby in birth crisis.

How do you imagine the birth?

While there are two ways for your baby to enter the world, there are a number of different environments where your baby can be delivered:

- At home with a midwife
- In a selected hospital or birthing clinic with an obstetrician or midwife
- In a hospital theatre, via a planned (elective) or unplanned (urgent) C-section

When considering your birth preference, remember that you have an innate ability to give birth naturally. Believing in yourself and your ability will result in a higher likelihood of a natural delivery.

Also, you must realise that a C-section is major surgery. It requires a 10 cm incision through your abdomen and uterine wall, and a full recovery period afterwards. You won't be able to drive for a few weeks. As with any surgical procedure there are myriad possible complications. A C-section is not necessarily the safer option for a healthy baby and mom in an uncomplicated delivery.

Step 2: Understand South African realities

Once you understand your preference there are factors you need to be aware of that will most likely affect your choice.

Your birth preference may be affected by your medical scheme

Medical schemes do not necessarily reimburse all of the costs of pregnancy care and delivery. Find out what your policy includes. To qualify for medical aid cover, you must have been a member before conception.

If you do not belong to a medical scheme and cannot afford private care, you will probably give birth in a state facility with a midwife, where you are less likely to have a C-section.

World's highest C-section rate

At 75 per cent, private hospitals in South Africa have one of the highest C-section rates in the world: three out of four obstetrician-led births are C-sections. In contrast, four out of five births with a private midwife are natural deliveries. Most are in private hospitals.

The statistics make the reality clear. You are most likely to have a natural birth with a private midwife or an obstetrician with a low C-section rate.

There are some obstetricians who have reasonable C-section rates, but many have exceptionally high rates, even as high as 100 per cent. If you choose an obstetrician with a high C-section rate your chance of a natural birth is extremely low (see below: What is a normal C-section rate?).

The impact of litigation

As a result of increased litigation, caregivers have to pay expensive litigation insurance. This increased financial burden may cause caregivers to be more cautious and have a lower threshold to perform a C-section, which might be more predictable.

Convenience and efficiency

If you and your caregiver prioritise control and predictability, you are more likely to have a planned C-section, which enables doctors to organise hospital and office time, and reduce evening, night, weekend and holiday call-outs.

Your expectations

If you insist on having your own obstetrician deliver your baby you are more likely to have a C-section. Obstetricians like weekends and holidays too! If your obstetrician is not on call when you go into labour, a locum or backup doctor will deliver your baby.

Interventions during labour have a knock-on effect

Statistics show that you are more likely to have a C-section if you experience an intervention during labour. Common interventions include inductions, epidurals and continuous foetal monitoring. An intervention may be necessary, but it reduces your chance of a natural birth.

> ### WHAT IS A NORMAL C-SECTION RATE?
>
> Our private health-care system has one of the highest C-section rates in the world (75 per cent). In America, the figure is 33 per cent. In the United Kingdom and northern Europe, it ranges from 10 to 20 per cent. The World Health Organization recommends a C-section rate of 10 to 15 births in 100. Studies indicate that if more than 20 out of 100 babies are delivered by C-section **the risks outweigh the benefits**. The high C-section rate in the private sector may suggest that the health of the mother and the baby is not always the priority.

Step 3: Choose your caregiver with sense

Once you have decided on a natural birth or elective C-section, and you are informed about the realities in South Africa, you must choose a midwife or an obstetrician. If you do not already have a valued caregiver, interview prospective candidates.

You must find someone with whom you can build a relationship. If there is a relationship of trust, you will know that your caregiver has your interests at heart and you will not feel cheated out of the birth you were hoping for if the delivery does not go to plan. Be flexible and relaxed. Births do not always go as hoped for.

OPTION 1: INDEPENDENT MIDWIFE

- For normal and uncomplicated births, midwives are as qualified as obstetricians and are frequently more passionate about delivering babies vaginally.
- Midwives can deliver at home, in a supported hospital or a private birthing clinic.
- If you are under a midwife's care, it is necessary to have a backup obstetrician.
- In a high-risk pregnancy (multiples, a diabetic mother), referral to an obstetrician is necessary.
- Some medical schemes, hospitals and obstetricians do not support private midwives.

OPTION 2: OBSTETRICIAN

- An obstetrician can manage all pregnancies and births.
- An obstetrician will liaise with hospital-employed midwives who monitor and support you during labour; he or she will then deliver your baby, vaginally or by C-section if necessary.
- You may ask an obstetrician to be backup doctor if you choose a midwife as your caregiver.
- If your preference is a natural delivery, ask about the obstetrician's C-section rate, which vary from 32 to 100 per cent.

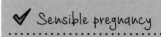

Sensible pregnancy

Find out ...
- Do you have matching philosophies around birth?
- Is there room for shared decision-making?
- How much time does the caregiver allow for questions?
- What is the C-section rate of the caregiver/hospital?
- Does he or she display:
  - Compassion: will the caregiver address your concerns?
  - Common courtesy: does your caregiver include your partner in the consultations?

WHEN FALLING PREGNANT IS TOUGH

After Jenny's rapid climb up the corporate ladder and six years of marriage, her biological clock began ticking and the moment she focused on this it was as if she could hear nothing else. She assumed that she would simply fall pregnant when she went off the pill but this did not happen. As the months went by, Jenny would hold her breath around the day when her period should come. Would this be her month? Could she possibly be pregnant?

She thought nothing could be worse until she actually fell pregnant but lost the baby after six weeks. This emotional roller coaster was almost too much to bear.

If you are battling to fall pregnant or have suffered the loss of a baby, you will be familiar with the cycles of hope, anxiety, elation and grief. If you have put off falling pregnant for career or personal reasons, you may experience a sense of regret that you did not embark on this journey earlier. As each month passes, your sense of determination will increase and after a while falling pregnant may feel like an obsession, with little else occupying your mind. It is a very tough emotional journey.

Your caregiver

Choosing and trusting your fertility specialist is very important. You may find that, as you progress on the fertility journey, you hear about other 'better' caregivers or alternate solutions. Because your fertility specialist will build a picture over time, he or she is often more likely to find the right solution for you than if you regularly swap specialists.

Fertility treatment is expensive and in your search for a solution you may be exploited by people with promises of a solution. Remember that you are more vulnerable and desperate than you have ever been, so before heeding any advice to swap caregivers or try a new solution, do your research and be selective about whom you consult for fertility treatment.

Natural ways to increase fertility

- Weight loss in obese women does improve fertility rates. Conversely, women who are significantly underweight have a better chance of conceiving if they eat more healthily.
- Antioxidants (present in certain multivitamins, e.g. StaminoGro) have been linked to improved fertility.
- Acupuncture and reflexology are used and may assist in reducing stress, although there is no evidence that they increase pregnancy rates per se.

Fertility treatment

It is considered normal for a couple to take up to one year to conceive and normally no intervention would be considered before this.

- If you are over 37, you should consider consulting your obstetrician earlier (after six months).
- If your cycle is irregular three months after stopping contraception you should seek medical advice.
- If you have not conceived after a year of unprotected intercourse, it is appropriate to seek medical help.

Investigation covers three areas: to check that the semen quality is adequate (semen analysis), to confirm that the woman is ovulating, and to confirm that the fallopian tubes aren't blocked and there are no physical problems. An obstetrician can assess a couple and perform most of these tests. Referral to a fertility specialist may be necessary for treatment beyond this.

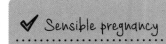

✔ Sensible pregnancy

Other options
Never lose sight of the fact that conception is unpredictable and no statistics can be completely accurate. Other options that should be considered by a couple who can't conceive, are surrogacy, the use of donor eggs or sperm and adoption.

LOSS

Losing a baby through miscarriage, termination due to foetal anomalies, late pregnancy loss, stillbirth or death, will result in enormous emotional pain and suffering. Even if you have not yet fallen pregnant, you may experience a sense of loss each time your period arrives.

Each woman will experiences this loss differently, depending on her age, how long she has been trying to fall pregnant, how many rounds of fertility treatment she has gone through, or simply the financial burden of treatment.

The way in which loss is processed is different for each individual and is not necessarily sequential. For many, there is an overwhelming sense of disbelief and shock. You may also feel angry about the perceived unfairness of your situation, or guilt at something you may or may not have

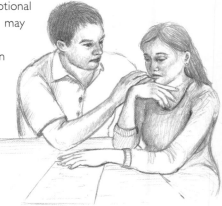

done to cause the loss. There may be periods of depression and despair, but bear in mind that it does get easier. In time you will find hope as you start the process over.

Your partner

Fertility problems put enormous strain on your relationship. Not only is the emotional rollercoaster of loss and disappointment taxing, but the flood of hormones and medical interventions are also likely to make you fractious and irritable. Conflict about the financial cost of treatment may aggravate the strain.

It is critical that you and your partner do not allow blame or guilt to affect your relationship. Focusing on whose fault it is, is not helpful in any way.

Protect your relationship:

• Do not blame each other.
• Consider your financial position from the start – how will you afford this?
• Work out whether you are both on the same page with how far you want to go with fertility treatment.
• Discuss how important it is for each of you to have a child.
• Look after yourselves and each other.

The esSense of falling pregnant

⚬ You can fall pregnant safely after stopping most contraceptives. It is wise to wait for your first real period after stopping the pill as this makes estimating a due date easier.

⚬ Check that you are immune to German measles, chicken-pox, whooping cough and this season's flu before falling pregnant.

⚬ Start using a folic acid supplement when you decide to stop contraception or before going off the pill if you take oral contraceptives.

⚬ Certain STDs are dangerous for your baby's health; make sure you know your status and discuss this with your doctor.

⚬ Choosing your caregiver needs very careful consideration as it has a direct bearing on where and how you will deliver.

⚬ Infertility brings cycles of hope, anxiety, elation and grief. You will need support through this process.

Section 2

CHAPTER 5

0–8 weeks

A 40-week pregnancy is calculated from the first day of your last menstrual period (LMP), which is two weeks before ovulation. So for the first two weeks of pregnancy you are actually not pregnant. By the time you miss your first period, you are considered to be four weeks pregnant and by the time you see your baby's heartbeat on the first scan, you will be six weeks pregnant. The first eight weeks of pregnancy pass rapidly and with few problems for most. But in these weeks your baby is developing at an incredible rate.

CONFIRMING PREGNANCY

Am I pregnant?
It is amazing how often women 'just know' that they are pregnant. There is an awareness of changes and subtle early signs. These vary from one woman to the next and may include the following:

TENDER BREASTS
Breast tenderness is usually the earliest symptom that you may become aware of. Your nipples may be especially sensitive and darken slightly. While this is quite common when you are premenstrual, if it is worsening, think pregnancy. Your breasts may also increase in size.

BLOATING
You may find that you feel 'fatter' or bloated and may even experience a little constipation.

MISSED PERIOD
It is quite normal for a menstrual cycle to vary by two days, but if your period is more than three or four days overdue, you may be pregnant.

FATIGUE

Extreme fatigue is a common early pregnancy sign. This often goes hand in hand with nausea – starting at five to six weeks from your last period and only improving around 12 to 14 weeks.

HEIGHTENED SENSE OF SMELL AND NAUSEA

A heightened sense of smell may result in feelings of nausea. This can start around five to six weeks and resolve around 12 weeks. It may be mild – no more than a gnawing hunger pain, but it may be severe enough cause vomiting, significant weight loss and hospitalisation. It is usually worst on an empty stomach. Sometimes it manifests as an aversion to or dislike of certain foods or odours.

INCREASED URINATION

As your kidneys produce more urine and there is pressure on your bladder, you may need to urinate more often.

Pregnancy tests

If you are experiencing any or all of these signs, particularly if you have missed your period, it is time to do a pregnancy test.

URINE TESTS

Urine tests are **very** accurate at diagnosing pregnancy. They detect the beta-hCG hormone as early as the time of the missed period (see illustration on the right).

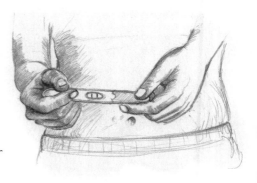

Purchase a pregnancy test from your pharmacy and carry out the test according to instructions ideally first thing in the morning. A positive test is almost certainly correct. Should the test be negative, it is worth repeating in a few days' time and testing your urine first thing in the morning when it is concentrated and the beta-hCG easier to detect.

BLOOD TESTS

They also test for betaHCG and have two functions – they can tell you *if* you are pregnant and *how far* your pregnancy is by measuring the actual level of betaHCG. Blood tests are able to detect pregnancy at the time of implantation – 6 to 12 days after fertilisation.

ULTRASOUND SCAN

Ultrasound scans can detect pregnancy once there is a sac visible in the uterine cavity – at about five weeks after your LMP. A scan will confirm that your pregnancy is viable once a heartbeat can be detected – usually at six to seven weeks from LMP. In addition to diagnosing pregnancy, ultrasound is important to confirm that the pregnancy is in the uterus, not an ectopic pregnancy, and also to see how many foetuses there are. In early pregnancy, a transvaginal ultrasound – where an ultrasound probe is placed in the vagina – is

> ### Making sense
> . . . .
> An **ectopic pregnancy** is a pregnancy outside of the uterus, most frequently in the fallopian tube.

often performed. With modern technology, an adequate view might be obtained scanning trans-abdominally (from the tummy) if the bladder is full.

Working out your due date

The average human pregnancy is 40 weeks or 280 days from the first day of the LMP. It is normal for a woman to go into labour from 37 completed weeks, up to 42 weeks from the LMP. Only 4–5 per cent of babies actually arrive on their due date.

To work out your expected date of delivery (EDD), add seven days to the date of your LMP and subtract three months. This is when your baby will be due (Naegele's rule). This method is accurate for women who have a 28-day menstrual cycle. The EDD will be earlier for women who have a shorter cycle, and later for women who have a longer cycle. There are a multitude of smartphone apps and calculators available on the internet to save you the maths.

MULTIPLE PREGNANCY

Early diagnosis of a multiple baby pregnancy is important. Because of fertility treatment and the increasing age at which many women have children, multiple pregnancies occur more frequently – in 2 to 3 per cent of births.

An ultrasound early on is the best time to establish whether the placenta and/or amniotic sacs are shared or separate. This has an enormous impact on how your pregnancy is managed.

If two different sperm fertilise two different eggs you will have non-identical (fraternal) twins. Each baby has her own sac and a separate placenta. This is the commonest form of twins. The likelihood of non-identical twins increases if there is a family history and varies enormously in different ethnic groups (much more prevalent in black South Africans than other race groups).

Identical twins occur when one zygote splits to form two embryos at around week 3 (one week after fertilisation). Some of these twins share one amniotic sac and the placenta. Other identical twins each have a separate amniotic sac but share a placenta.

Almost all pregnancy symptoms, including nausea and fatigue, are worse with a multiple pregnancy.

CARING FOR YOURSELF

From the moment you discover that you are pregnant, and for many even earlier, you will begin a journey of increased awareness of what you ingest. Studies have shown that more than 86 per cent of mothers will make at least three significant changes to their diet during the first and second trimester. This is a good time to reassess your diet and the choices you make around food:

• Limit processed carbohydrates.
• Do not eat foods that can cause infections.
• Do not drink alcohol.

Supplements

Even if you have a healthy diet, you need to take a folic acid supplement at this stage. Also eat foods rich in folic acid, including lentils, dried beans and peas, dark-green vegetables such as broccoli, spinach, okra and asparagus, and citrus fruit and juice.

It is not necessary to take additional iron yet.

Exercise

You can continue with whatever exercise you did prior to falling pregnant. Listen to your body and don't push yourself. If you are tired, tone it down or even skip a day. If you were not exercising before falling pregnant, start by doing something gentle and relaxing like taking a walk or swimming some pool laps.

Weight gain

You will want to be aware of how much weight you should gain based on whether you were under- or over-weight before falling pregnant (see p. 26). Weight gain can have a direct bearing on the health of your baby.

In the first eight weeks, you are unlikely to gain any weight. If you are feeling 'fat' already, it is more likely due to bloating and gas than actual weight gain. Some moms put on 500 g but if you have gained more than this, now is the time to establish healthy eating habits of regular small meals with lots of water to drink.

'Morning' sickness

Nausea can actually occur at any time, but is more common in the morning when our blood sugar is lower. Prepearing a small wake-up snack, e.g. some dry biscuits, natural grains (such as quinoa or oats), nuts and fruit to have before getting up may help you feel better.

Antenatal appointments

Antenatal appointments are regular visits to your midwife, doctor or obstetrician where you are given information, where your and your baby's wellbeing is monitored and your expectations of pregnancy and delivery are discussed.

FIRST VISIT

Schedule your first visit around 8 to 10 weeks from your last period, but before 12 weeks, so that there is adequate time to consider the various tests that are available, e.g. testing for Down's Syndrome. Ultrasound at this point is clear and the foetus is easily visible.

You should make an earlier appointment if there has been bleeding or pain, or if you have had an ectopic pregnancy before.

SUBSEQUENT APPOINTMENTS

Antenatal visits are usually scheduled approximately every four weeks, and more frequently in the last month of pregnancy. You will probably see your caregiver at 8, 12 to 13, 16, 20, 25, 28, 31, 34, 36, 38, 40 and 41 weeks.

BECOMING A MOM

Your emotional state in the first two months of pregnancy will be strongly influenced by how planned and wanted your baby is. If you have planned to fall pregnant you will be very excited and delighted by your new status. If you have previously miscarried or struggled to fall pregnant, you may find that your fear of loss overrides the positive emotions. If your pregnancy was a surprise, you may feel ambivalent about it.

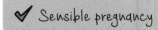 **Sensible pregnancy**

Calling your caregiver
Bleeding
Bleeding in pregnancy is abnormal, but not always associated with a bad outcome.

No need to call your caregiver
There may be spotting when the embryo buries itself into the lining of the uterus. This is called an implantation bleed and occurs about 10 days after conception, which is frequently around the time of the missed period. Bleeding after intercourse is due to contact with the tissues of the vagina and cervix, which have an increased blood supply in pregnancy.

Call your caregiver Ongoing or heavy bleeding (as heavy as a period) can be a sign of impending miscarriage or an ectopic pregnancy and should be investigated.

Pain
No need to call your caregiver
Slight discomfort and cramping, frequently experienced in early pregnancy, is nothing to worry about.

Call your caregiver Miscarriage is usually accompanied by significant period-like cramping. This and severe pain should be investigated. An ectopic pregnancy causes lower abdominal pain, often more severe on one side than the other, and might spread to the upper abdomen or be felt in the shoulders.

Weekly progress

WEEK	Your baby's development	Your changing body
1	This is the first week after your period. The egg that is destined to form a precious person is yet to be fertilised by your partner's sperm.	In the first week of 'pregnancy' fertilisation has not happened but your body is ready. The uterus wall is becoming nice and thick to provide the best environment for your baby to develop.
2	At the end of week 2, around 14 days after your last period, the egg is released from the ovary and begins its journey down the fallopian tube. At this time the mucus within your vagina is very liquid, perfect for millions of sperm to swim through to reach the egg, which is now situated within the fallopian tube.	You may feel more amorous and may experience ovulation pain on the day the egg is released.

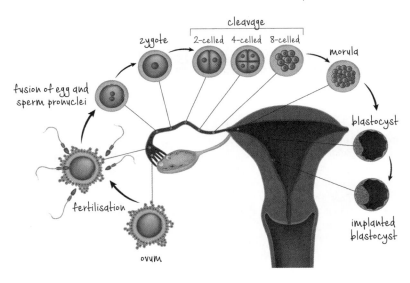

WEEK	Your baby's development	Your changing body
3	Within spilt seconds of a sperm fertilising the egg, the great division of cells begins, forming more and more cells. Within a couple of days the fertilised cell looks like a mulberry the size of a pinprick, containing all the genes that will code for every one of your baby's features – gender, hair colour, height and temperament. We call this stage the zygote. The zygote travels along the fallopian tube before moving to the uterus where, after about two days, it burrows into the uterine wall. This process, called implantation, occurs 7 to 12 days after fertilisation. If you are going to have identical twins, there is a good chance that the zygote will split to become two embryos this week or next.	Before you are even aware you are pregnant, your baby starts to form and your body begins to change. You may feel bloated and gassy this week owing to the increased progesterone. You may also spot as your baby implants in the uterus.

WEEK	Your baby's development	Your changing body
4	The zygote is now embedded in the uterine wall where your baby will grow for the next nine months. At this stage, the embryo gets its nourishment from a yolk sac, until the placenta can take over. To form the placenta, part of the mass of cells extends even deeper into the uterine wall and little finger-like projections bury in. It can take up to week 6 for the embryo to fully implant and until week 12 to develop a fully functioning, healthy placenta that will deliver oxygen and nutrients to and remove waste products from your baby for the next seven to eight months. The outer cells of the embryo fold into the middle of the ball of cells, like a finger pressing into a balloon, and this is the start of the formation of cells that form the spinal cord and the brain. Three layers develop at around this time: • The inner layer of cells will form your baby's organs. • The outer layer forms the skin, sensory organs and brain. • The middle layer will develop into the bones, muscles and blood and heart. Now your baby is called an embryo and is less than 3 mm long, yet her nervous system (brain and spine) and her circulatory system (heart and arteries) are already forming, preparing to get her moving and her heart pumping blood.	You will have missed your period this week and the release of hCG (the pregnancy hormone) may cause tender breasts and leave you feeling emotional. If you take a home pregnancy test this week, it may be positive.
5	Your baby is 3 mm long – around the size of an apple pip. She resembles a tadpole and her heart is actively forming, ready to start beating in the next week. Her brain and all the organs (kidneys, liver and intestines) are developing at this point while little buds for the arms and legs emerge. Your baby's first nerves for hearing start to develop. Until the foetus is embedded in the uterus it is unlikely to be affected by environmental factors such as alcohol or other teratogens.	Some moms feel no pregnancy symptoms yet, while for others the fatigue of pregnancy sets in. You may start to urinate frequently too.
6	Your baby's heart begins to beat. For the first few days the heartbeat is slow (around 60 beats per minute), but thereafter it reaches almost double your heart rate - around 170 beats per minute and slows to 110–160 by full term. Around this time, your baby's neural tube (brain and spine) will start to close. A baby whose neural tube does not close has *spina bifida*. Taking folic acid supplements has been shown to prevent this. Your baby is around 4 mm long now and her neck and face begin to form. Spots appear on the side of the head, which will develop into eyes, and the very first visual tissue can be seen.	Your hormones will make you sensitive and you may experience mood swings. Nausea often starts at around six weeks. You may only be aware of increased hunger, but nausea, at any time and not only in the morning, is frequent and vomiting is common. Brushing your teeth may trigger nausea and vomiting. Some women develop strong aversions to certain foods and smells.

WEEK	Your baby's development	Your changing body
7	Your baby measures 8 mm and starts to look like a baby now. Little arms and legs are developing as are her facial features. Ears start forming but your baby cannot yet hear. 　At 7½ weeks your baby's sense of touch begins to develop, first around the mouth and lips. At the same time, the hearing and movement system in the inner ear begins to form. Since this forms so early, it is a vulnerable sense and some illnesses like German measles can disrupt the development of hearing.	The *corpus luteum* in your ovary is already producing enormous amounts of oestrogen and progesterone resulting in the marvellous changes that occur in your body during pregnancy. You are aware of changes, such as breast tingling, pain and fullness.
8	Your baby's brain is rapidly growing and her spinal column is now closed, encasing the nerves that make up the spinal cord. Your baby is growing about one millimetre a day and is around 15 mm long now. Her little arms and legs are developing rapidly and start to move. Separate fingers and toes form but are still webbed. This is the first time that any foetal movement can be detected. 　Your baby's taste buds form and her palate and teeth are developing too. Veins can be seen through her paper-thin skin. 　At this stage of pregnancy brain cells develop at a rate of about 250 000 per minute and cells begin to migrate to the right area of the brain. This migration of brain cells to the appropriate place creates the platform for the development of all skills – walking, talking, relating to people and reasoning.	Although you are not showing yet, your uterus is bigger and presses on your bladder, causing you to urinate more often. Your breasts are tender and definitely look and feel bigger.

Things to do

- **Avoid toxins**. Alcohol, nicotine, all recreational drugs and many over-the-counter medications are toxic to your baby. Make the healthy choice to avoid all these hazards for your baby.
- **Take folic acid**. Start taking folic acid as soon as you are thinking about falling pregnant. This is vital for the formation of the spinal cord and for protection against certain malformations.
- **Consider what changes to make**. If you are going to make any big changes, such as a job, house or lifestyle changes to afford your baby, now is the time to think about it, if you haven't already.
- **Take a pregnancy test**. It's time to confirm that you are pregnant. Occasionally an early pregnancy test comes up as a false negative and needs to be taken again if your period is late.
- **Book an appointment to see your caregiver**. When your home pregnancy test is positive it is time to make an appointment with a pregnancy caregiver. Chapter 4 (see p. 45) will guide you in choosing the caregiver who will best suit your birth preferences. Your caregiver will also do a urine test, check your blood pressure and confirm your due date.
- **Have an ultrasound**. An ultrasound will confirm your pregnancy and how many babies you are carrying.

✔ Sensible pregnancy

When not to worry
Many moms worry about what they did before they knew they were pregnant and how their lifestyle choices such as drinking alcohol or smoking affect their baby. Rest assured that teratogens (poisons for the foetus) ingested before the foetus embeds in the uterus (week 4–6) and a placenta develops are very unlikely to affect your baby.

Frequently asked questions

IS SEX SAFE?

Intercourse is completely safe in a normal pregnancy. Be honest and open with your partner about how you both feel about intercourse – you might not feel comfortable at different stages in pregnancy; your partner might have concerns about safety (see p 34).

HINTS FOR THE OTHER HALF

Depending on whether your pregnancy is planned and whether you feel ready to become a parent, this may be an exciting or unsettling time. Although *your* body is not changing, and your life won't be changing much for many months' time, you have the challenge and gift of time to prepare your physical world, your relationship and your mind for the arrival of your baby.

- Stay connected to your partner, ask how she feels, listen to her feelings and thoughts, and respond with yours. Be honest.
- Don't stress if the pregnancy doesn't feel real for you yet – this is common for expectant dads.
- Chat to your dad and your friends with children about becoming a father.
- An excellent book to read is *Fab Dad – A man's guide to fathering* by Paul Kerton.
- Show you care by joining your partner in eating healthily, abstaining from alcohol to keep her company, and not smoking in her presence.
- She may be nauseous and low on energy in these early weeks of the pregnancy, and irritability is common. Show empathy and support her rather than immediately withdrawing.
- Your partner may find it difficult to prepare food due to nausea; if you haven't been helping with meal preparation until now, take over in the kitchen.

The esSense of 0–8 weeks

- Your first symptom is likely to be tender or sore breasts, followed by feeling bloated. These may occur before you miss your first period, which is the first firm sign of pregnancy.

- Seven to twelve days after conception (week 3-4), the embryo embeds in the wall of your uterus and you may spot a little on that day.

- You are unlikely to have gained any weight yet but may feel bloated, which can make your clothes feel a little tight. Some women begin to feel nauseous as early as week 6.

- By week 7, your baby's organs are forming rapidly, her heart is beating and her arm and leg buds are developing. She can feel touch to her mouth area and her eyes begin to form.

- Take a pregnancy test after you miss your period and book your first antenatal visit for eight weeks after your last menstrual period (LMP).

CHAPTER 6

9–13 weeks

For many moms this second part of the first trimester is not the most pleasant. Your hormones kick in and leave you in no doubt that you are pregnant. Fatigue, nausea and general aches and pains characterise this stage.

CARING FOR YOURSELF

Dealing with nausea

You no doubt have the greatest intentions to eat healthy balanced meals, yet the constant nausea and, for some, the vomiting make it impossible to stick to a healthy meal plan all the time. Nausea tends to be more severe in first pregnancies or if you're carrying more than one baby. Most women who experience nausea notice a dramatic improvement after the first trimester – at roughly 13 weeks. But for some the nausea and vomiting continue beyond the first trimester.

Everyone responds to food differently – most women can tolerate light and relatively bland foods, like yoghurt, cereal and fruit. Fruit smoothies are a popular choice with women suffering from morning sickness. Stick to foods that you can tolerate; these often include fruit, nuts, fresh salads and vegetables. Animal proteins and excessively fatty foods may be problematic for some moms. If you are really struggling to stomach food, a commercially available pregnancy shake may be useful to keep you nourished and stabilise blood sugar. Listen to your body to determine what's right for you.

Follow these simple steps to **relieve nausea and vomiting**:
- Eat small, light meals or snacks at frequent intervals.
- Before getting out of bed in the morning, eat a couple of cream crackers or a piece of dry toast (see p. 54).
- Have a small snack at bedtime or when you wake up to go to the bathroom in the night.
- Avoid greasy, rich, fatty and spicy foods.
- Suck on hard sweets or ginger pieces.
- Because you lose fluids when vomiting, it is important to take in enough liquids. Try sucking on ice chips or ice lollies. Drink frequent small sips of water instead of a whole glass of water all at once. Some women find that small sips of ginger ale or peppermint tea relieve their symptoms.

✔ Sensible pregnancy

When to call your caregiver

Throwing up several times a day may make it difficult for you to retain adequate fluids, which is a health concern for you and your baby. Call your doctor or midwife if:

- you have not been able to keep liquids down for more than one day;
- you're vomiting blood, which may appear bright red or look like black coffee granules;
- you lose more than 1 kg;
- you have vomited more than four times in one day;
- you notice that your urine is dark and concentrated.

Hyperemesis Gravidarum, excessive nausea and vomiting in early pregnancy, can lead to dehydration, electrolyte imbalance and weight loss. This needs to be treated with medication, and hospitalisation for intravenous fluids is often necessary.

Supplements

Continue to take your folic acid supplement. It is still not necessary to take an iron supplement. Zinc, selenium and vitamin C can be added to help boost your immune system, which is often compromised in the first trimester, because your body uses so much energy for your developing baby.

Exercise

You may be feeling really tired and not be able to manage as much exercise as you used to. Listen to your body and be guided by how much energy you have.

Weight gain

It is advisable to gain 1–2 kg in the first trimester but this will vary from woman to woman. You may actually lose weight during this trimester, especially if you are struggling to eat and keep food down. Be mindful of excessive weight loss and speak to your caregiver regarding supplements should you be concerned.

If your weight gain is significant (more than 3 kg) you may be eating too much. Remember to eat healthily, not for two!

MULTIPLE PREGNANCY

As there is an increased risk for complications, a multiple pregnancy requires increased monitoring and specialist care. The risk depends a lot on the type of twins (see p. 53). Determining whether each baby is in his own sac is relatively easy early on, therefore a specialist ultrasound at this time is strongly recommended.

If you choose to, the combined test (see below), can also be used to assess the risk of chromosome abnormality for each foetus.

Constipation

Hormones are responsible for early-pregnancy constipation as progesterone slows down the peristaltic motion of the muscles of the intestines. Because digestion slows down, your body is able to draw more water from your food, leaving a harder mass to eliminate. If you are uncomfortable, consult your caregiver, as you need to prevent piles. Eating a well-balanced diet with lots of fruit and vegetables and drinking sufficient water will also help (see pp. 27–28).

Antenatal appointments

Through your pregnancy, depending on your risk factors and stage of pregnancy, you will be advised to have certain tests – from simple urine tests, to blood tests, and possibly a more invasive amniocentesis.

BLOOD TESTS

Routine antenatal blood tests, recommended for all pregnant women, include:

- **Anaemia** Your haemoglobin level will be tested to detect anaemia. Iron deficiency is the most common cause of anaemia in pregnancy and is easily treated with iron supplements. There are other, less common causes which will be investigated, if necessary.
- **Blood group** It is essential to know your blood group, determined by a test. If your blood group is rhesus negative, you will be tested for the presence of antibodies, as these might cross the placenta and cause anaemia and other complications for your baby.

TESTS IN PREGNANCY

A **screening test** determines your or your baby's risk of suffering from a condition. It is expressed as a chance of 1 in 'so many', e.g. a 1 in 1 000 chance of your baby's having Down's Syndrome.

A **diagnostic test** tells you whether you do or do not have a condition.

- **Glucose** Your body may not process glucose as effectively as before pregnancy and glucose in your urine may be normal. Your caregiver will determine if you require screening for diabetes. Some obstetricians prefer all pregnant women to have glucose testing; others only test if there are certain risk factors (e.g. obesity, family history).
- **Infections** Some infections that can be transferred to your baby may cause problems. You will be wise to consider tests for these early in pregnancy. They include immunity to infectious diseases such as rubella (German measles), and STDs such as syphilis, hepatitis B, and HIV (see Chapter 4, pp. 41–43).

OTHER TESTS
Testing for thyroid levels and for immunity to toxoplasmosis is not routine and is only recommended when appropriate.

Down's Syndrome and other chromosomal abnormalities
A woman's risk of having a baby with Down's Syndrome increases with age, but age alone is a very poor predictor of risk. At this point in your pregnancy, you therefore need to make a decision regarding a screening test for Down's Syndrome (trisomy 21). Down's Syndrome cannot be diagnosed with certainty with an ultrasound scan. There are three screening tests and two diagnostic tests.

Screening tests
The **Combined Test (or Nuchal Translucency or NT scan)** is performed between 11 weeks and 13 weeks and 6 days. There are three parts to this test:
- An ultrasound expert will calculate your risk based on the thickness of the tissue behind the neck of the foetus (the nuchal fold) and the presence of a nasal bone.
- Your age will be considered.
- A blood sample will be taken between 10 and 13 weeks to measure beta-hCG and PAPP-A levels.

The **Triple (or Quadruple) Test** is another screening test for trisomy 21. It is less accurate than the combined test, but can be performed between 15 and 20 weeks. It calculates risk according to maternal age and levels of beta-hCG, AFP and oestriol (and can also include inhibin-A) in the blood.

The **Non-invasive Prenatal Test (NIPT)** detects minute amounts of DNA from the foetus in the mother's blood stream. This is a screening test, not a diagnostic test, but is very accurate. The test is expensive and does not replace the Combined Test.

Diagnostic tests
If the risk is high, you may want to consider further diagnostic testing by means of amniocentesis, or chorionic villous sampling (CVS). Both methods are done under ultrasound guidance by passing a needle through

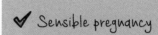
✔ Sensible pregnancy
....

Making the right decision
You may find it tough to make a decision about testing. Some people choose to test so that they can be prepared for a child with Down's Syndrome, or because they would consider termination of pregnancy should this be diagnosed. Amniocentesis carries a risk to the foetus. If termination is not an option for you, consider carefully whether you want to do the screening test at all.

A lot more information than just your risk of trisomy 21 is obtained with the Combined Test, but this can be obtained later at the 20-week scan. Make sure that an accredited professional performs these ultrasound scans. The measurements are very precise, and decisions made according to the results are profound.

the mother's abdomen to obtain a sample of either amniotic fluid or placenta. You have to understand that there is a small risk (1 in 100 in expert hands) of either test resulting in a miscarriage.

BECOMING A MOM

You will be adjusting to the idea of being a mom if you have known for a month that you are pregnant. It is time to start thinking about how your emotional state affects your baby.

Stress in pregnancy does affect your baby:

- Experiencing a moderate amount of stress which you generally feel you can manage, will not harm your baby. Acute, short-lived surges of stress hormones are usually transient and do not have a negative effect on your baby. He feels the stress but the recovery after the stress may accelerate development and contribute to his ability to self-regulate and long-term resilience.
- If your stress is on-going, uncontrolled and interpersonal, we call it toxic stress and this can have negative consequences for your baby's development, growth and ability to regulate stress in the long term. Now is the time to make changes.

Coping with stress

If your baby is enduring long periods of stress you need to deal with it and make changes to your lifestyle:

- Talk to a caregiver or counsellor. Often, just sharing the load is enough.
- Seek non-judgemental support – someone who cares and will not express an opinion that stresses you further.
- Change anything that is within your control.
- If you cannot change the situation, you need to change the way you see it.

Weekly progress

WEEK	Your baby's development	Your changing body
9	Your baby is now about 2 cm long – the size of an olive. Until now, the human baby looks like almost all animal embryos. Now the tail disappears and he starts to look like a little person. His arms are growing longer and elbows begin to form. Your baby's muscles start to develop and, although you can't yet feel the movements, your baby is moving a lot. A huge amount is happening in his brain – his brain cells are forming and migrating to the right place, and start to branch out and connect to form early brain pathways. Your baby now has a mouth and tongue and his taste buds are forming on his tongue. His nostrils form and nerves for the sense of smell start to develop.	Your uterus is now the size of a grapefruit and you may experience some weight gain, with your clothes feeling a little tight.

WEEK	Your baby's development	Your changing body
10	At 3 cm long your baby now looks like a tiny human with forward-facing eyes and all his fingers and toes. All major organs are in place but not fully formed or functional yet. Your baby starts to move his hands, taking them to his mouth and face. In this week the teeth buds and bones are also forming. At this stage we can see the vestibular canals in the inner ear, which will form the sensory system that perceives movement and creates a base for coordination. Your baby is preparing to be a mover and shaker. His taste buds continue to form. Your baby's optic nerve for vision starts to develop, as well as his eyelids, although they will be closed for the next few months of pregnancy.	Nausea and morning sickness continue to plague many women. In addition to the bloating and fatigue, these symptoms are the bane of the first trimester. Your breasts are likely to enlarge further and you may notice a road map of veins over your chest area.
11	Your baby is perfectly formed, including all his organs, and we now call the embryo a foetus. His ears are in the right place and all 10 fingers and 10 toes are actively moving and can feel touch. His hair follicles and his sex organs are developing. Now that the spinal cord is completely formed and functional, your baby's reflexes begin to develop. All movements at this stage are reflexive (not intentional). The startle reflex is one of the first reflexes and emerges this week. Your baby's mouth opens and closes. Measured from the top of his head to his bum, he is about 4.1 cm long – the size of a small lime. 	You may feel like you are starting to show but most of your tummy distension is due to bloating, gas and increased bowel contents as you may be constipated due to the progesterone, which slows down digestion. Vaginal discharge will increase and will be present throughout your pregnancy. At around this time, the placenta takes over hormone production from the *corpus luteum*. During pregnancy, a woman produces as much oestrogen as a non-pregnant woman would in 150 years. It's no wonder that the changes are profound.

WEEK	Your baby's development	Your changing body
12	The movement reflexes you will see at birth, such as the sucking, grasp and startle reflexes, are emerging in earnest. Your baby may start to hiccup occasionally, although you won't yet feel these little movements. Your baby's sense of touch is developing; within the next two weeks, towards the end of the first trimester, he can perceive touch on his entire body, except the top of his head, which we believe remains insensitive until just after birth – maybe so your little one doesn't feel the squeeze through the birth canal. Your baby is not conscious of pain or touch until later in the second trimester when the tracts for touch connect to the conscious brain. Your baby is 5,8 cm long and his head is about half the size of his body.	The end of the first trimester is in sight and, for most, the difficult early symptoms of pregnancy such as fatigue and nausea start to abate. The risk of miscarriage decreases markedly and most people choose this time to share the good news with family and friends. The uterine wall thickens and the uterus fills the pelvis. As the foetus grows, the pregnancy sac fills the uterine cavity. Although the uterus is confined to the pelvic cavity until 12 weeks, your tummy becomes fuller, and the waist circumference increases.
13	Your baby is about 7,5 cm long and the organs are actively developing. His lungs begin to form and he will perform 'breathing actions' as he prepares to take that first breath in six months' time. The other organs are also becoming functional – the liver secretes bile and the kidneys release urine to his bladder, which discharges it into the amniotic fluid when he urinates. The smell system is ready to start perceiving smells but doesn't function yet owing to a plug of tissue in the nostrils. Your baby's cochlea (hearing apparatus) looks like an adult's and connects through the auditory nerve to the brain. Your baby is developing fingerprints! What a miracle of development – in 13 short weeks a baby human being has formed inside you.	You may see changes in pigmentation – not only do your nipples and the areola (the area around the nipple) become darker, you may also start to develop dark patches on your skin. A dark line on your tummy, the *linea nigra*, may start to form. The blood vessels of the vulva and vagina become engorged and appear purple. The breast changes of pregnancy persist although the tenderness usually lessens.

Things to do

- **Plan where you want to give birth.** It's time to start thinking of where you want to have your baby: at home or in hospital. Discuss these plans with your caregiver and determine if he or she can accommodate your wishes. Most doctors will not deliver a baby at home, but some are prepared to provide hospital backup for a midwife, should you choose a home delivery.
- **Buy maternity clothes.** Try to stick to soft, comfortable fabrics. Leggings are a great choice as they can stretch over your growing curves.
- **Decide on screening tests.** You will have a big check-up at around this time. You will be scanned and may have blood taken. At this check-up, you will need to decide whether to test for Down's Syndrome.
- **Take pregnancy supplements.** Don't forget to keep taking your pregnancy vitamins and other supplements as prescribed by your caregiver.
- **Moisturise your skin.** Start using a cream or oil that helps to prevent stretch marks by keeping your skin soft and supple.

Frequently asked questions

When shall we tell?

There is no right or wrong time to tell friends or family that you are pregnant. Some of us will blurt it out as soon as a double line appears on the pregnancy test, while others are more discreet and will wait until the pregnancy is quite advanced.

Early miscarriage is common – about one in six pregnancies miscarry spontaneously before 12 weeks. Many couples choose to wait until 12 weeks before announcing their pregnancy. Once you have had an ultrasound scan and the presence of the heartbeat has been confirmed, the risk of miscarriage is much lower.

If you choose to test for chromosomal abnormality, you might choose to wait for these results before sharing the news of your pregnancy.

Remember that, should things go wrong, close friends or family will be your support. These are the people you might tell earlier than others.

HINTS FOR THE OTHER HALF

- Help your partner feel good about herself, as the changes in her body during pregnancy may leave her feeling unattractive. Express appreciation for the sacrifices she is making to grow and nurture your baby.
- Tell her what qualities you love in her that you hope your baby inherits. (Don't mention the bits you hope your baby doesn't get from her –not even as a joke!)
- Accompany her to the 12-week scan and ask her if she wants you to accompany her to all the visits. Being included helps you feel involved and is exciting, and helps your partner feel supported.
- Hopefully her nausea and fatigue/ irritability will improve by the end of this first trimester.

The esSense of 9–13 weeks

- Your placenta fully develops and takes over providing the hormones for pregnancy.

- Physical niggles increase – nausea, bloating and sore breasts are the order of the day. You will notice your breasts enlarge, your nipples get darker and the veins to your breasts are more noticeable – your perfect body is preparing to nourish your newborn.

- By the end of the first trimester you may have gained 1-2 kg.

- The first trimester is a critical time for development – your little one starts to move. The movements are all reflexes and not intentional. The touch receptors are fully developed and the organs and nerves for vision, hearing and smell are starting to form.

- You will see your caregiver once during this stage – usually before 12 weeks, and at this appointment will make decisions on which screening tests you wish to have.

CHAPTER 7

14–18 weeks

As the second trimester gets under way, most women experience increased energy, less nausea and that famous pregnancy glow that sets in for the next few months. Not everyone experiences the same glow; feelings of vulnerability and dependence may dampen the positive feelings you would otherwise bask in.

CARING FOR YOURSELF

The second trimester is a great time to establish healthy eating habits and to really focus on nourishing your body and your growing baby. The focus is on eating unrefined starches that are naturally occurring in nature, e.g. vegetables, fresh seasonal fruit, and some complex grains like quinoa, millet, spelt and stone-ground flour. Aim to include something raw, such as fresh fruit or salad, with each meal.

Supplements

Now that you are less queasy, you can start taking a comprehensive antenatal supplement that includes iron. Try to choose one with non-constipating or gentle iron.

Exercise

The huge burst of energy of this trimester means you can continue your normal exercise routine. It is a good idea to add some core-strengthening exercises like yoga or Pilates.

Weight gain

If this is your first pregnancy, you may not be showing yet, but subsequent pregnancies are often noticed earlier as the abdominal wall muscles are looser and allow the uterus to protrude easily. If you lost weight with morning sickness in the first trimester, you will start to regain this and then gain some more. You may be gaining between 1 and 2 kg a month now, reaching 2,5 to 5 kg total weight gain by the end of this stage, depending on your pre-pregnancy weight.

Weight gained in the first half of pregnancy comes from increased blood volume and fat deposits. This fat is accumulated to provide energy later in the pregnancy and to meet the demands of breast-feeding. Weight gained in the second half of pregnancy is mostly from the baby, placenta, amniotic fluid and fluid accumulated in the mother's tissues.

Morning sickness

For most women, morning sickness has passed and they can start to enjoy food again. However, there is a small percentage of moms who experience morning sickness right through the second trimester or

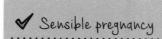

Sensible pregnancy

How often should you be weighed?
You may be weighed at every visit, although some caregivers advocate **not** weighing pregnant women as it causes anxiety and doesn't often provide any additional benefit. New guidelines recommend an initial assessment of BMI, but **not** regular weighing unless it is indicated – for obese or underweight mothers, or if you have gestational diabetes.

even longer. If you are one of these unlucky moms and you are not gaining weight, you need to seek help in order to provide sufficient nourishment for your growing baby.

Constipation

Constipation is another unwelcome but normal pregnancy change.

The muscular activity of the bowel wall is reduced and the 'transit time' of the bowel contents is slower, allowing for more water to be reabsorbed resulting in a firmer stool.

Regular exercise, adequate fluid intake and increased fibre intake (fruit and vegetables) will help. Despite these, constipation often needs treating. Avoid stimulatory laxatives; rather ask your caregiver to recommend a stool softener such as ispaghula, lactulose or polyethylene glycol (Movicol).

MULTIPLE PREGNANCY

You will have more frequent visits with your obstetrician; use these to discuss what troubles you, and what can be done. Be realistic regarding your own expectations about work and activity.

If each baby has her own placenta, you should have antenatal visits at least every four weeks until 32 weeks, and then every two weeks. Mothers of twins who share a placenta, will usually have two-weekly visits, and require two-weekly scans.

Antenatal appointments

At each antenatal visit, your caregiver will assess you physically, find out how you are coping and feeling, and also address any questions you may have. Your urine will be tested, blood pressure measured, abdomen examined, and you may be weighed.

Urine test

Your urine will be tested for:
- glucose, an indicator of gestational (pregnancy) diabetes;
- protein, to exclude preeclampsia or kidney disease;
- signs of urinary tract (bladder) infection which will be indicated by a positive result for white cells and nitrates on a dipstick test

Blood pressure

Your blood pressure will be measured to detect high blood pressure and preeclampsia. Blood pressure during pregnancy is usually lower than normal, until the last month of pregnancy, when it returns to normal pre-pregnancy levels. This low blood pressure can aggravate tiredness and increases the likelihood of fainting, or feeling faint, particularly when standing up quickly.

Abdominal examination

Your abdomen will be examined to assess the size of your uterus, and later how your baby is lying. Your caregiver will assess the amount of amniotic fluid by examining the abdomen, and also if there is any unusual tenderness.

Your baby's growth and the amount of amniotic fluid, is measured in centimetres using a tape measure, from the upper level of the uterus (the *fundus*) to the pubic bone (*symphysis pubis*). This is the

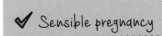 Sensible pregnancy
. . . .
When to call your caregiver
Bleeding in pregnancy always needs to be investigated.

Severe period like-pains must be looked into.

On-going vomiting and nausea ares unusual at this time and you should mention it to your doctor (see Chapter 6).

symphysis–fundal height. The measurement is plotted on a graph to check that growth is in the normal range.

ULTRASOUND

An obstetrician who has an ultrasound machine may use this to measure foetal growth and amniotic fluid.

There is no harm in having an ultrasound scan at every visit and although you will probably enjoy them, it is not necessary to have one every time.

Be aware that when a quick scan is done, it just measures the heart beat and growth of your baby. In-depth details of normality are **not** assessed in these scans.

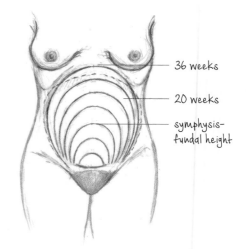

36 weeks

20 weeks

symphysis–fundal height

BECOMING A MOM

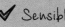 **Sensible pregnancy**

Recommended ultrasound scans

In a healthy pregnancy there is no reason to have a scan at every appointment but these are recommended:
- An early scan at 8 to 10 weeks to confirm your pregnancy and determine how far you are
- A combined test between 11 weeks and 13 weeks and 6 days to screen for Down's Syndrome, if you choose to do this test
- A detailed structural scan at 20 to 22 weeks

Other ultrasound scans might be indicated, for example if the placenta is low-lying, if your baby measures smaller or bigger than normal and in the case of multiple pregnancy.

Having reached the turning point of the 14-week mark means you can feel more secure about your pregnancy. If you have suffered losses before, you will probably only now allow yourself to get excited and tell people about your fabulous news. Your emotions are more stable and you may even experience feelings of elation in this trimester.

An area that may bring emotional turmoil is deciding about tests for birth defects that are usually performed around this time. Take the time to consider your options and risk profile. If you feel termination is not an option, you may question the value of the tests. A false positive or result that shows increased risk may also lead to undue stress and further procedures. It is stressful, no matter what your risk profile and how you decide to proceed. Discuss your options and feelings with your caregiver.

Making sense

Preggy brain

You *are* more forgetful during pregnancy and the first year of your baby's life. It's not a figment of your imagination. Research has shown that brain activity shifts to the emotional centres of the brain to prepare for bonding. It is also believed that a pregnant woman's ability to multitask and deal with more than one thing diminishes. This allows you to focus on your child's survival.

Weekly progress

WEEK	Your baby's development	Your changing body
14	Your baby is now the size of a lemon, around 9 cm long. She can swallow amniotic fluid and this week, her senses of smell and taste start to develop. As she gets older, she will swallow more vigorously when she tastes sweet flavours that you have ingested – already showing a preference for sweet over bitter. Because she can feel touch now, if she is touched on her cheek she will root (turn) towards the stimulus, and her sucking muscles are functioning. This is all in preparation for seeking out the breast for feeding. From 14 to 28 weeks, all visual structures will develop so your baby can see at birth. Even though the eyes begin to move around this time, your baby will only have more complex eye movements later in the second trimester. Sight is the least developed sense at birth because it gets very little practice in the womb, where it is dark without contrasting shapes and colours. Your baby's gender will become apparent this week and ovarian follicles begin forming if she is a girl.	At this stage, you will find your emotions starting to lift and your energy levels increase almost daily. You may have the odd bout of feeling ill or sensitivity to smell or tiredness, but soon these first trimester ailments will be gone too. Some women do take longer to feel relief from nausea and if you are still vomiting regularly you should chat to your caregiver.
15	Your baby is growing at an amazing rate, now measuring more than 10 cm. All her bones are forming and can be seen on ultrasound. Now that the little bones in the ear appear, your baby can start to hear and in the next few weeks will respond to sound. The formation of the hearing and balance organs (found in the ear) is at its most vulnerable at around this time. If your little one is exposed to certain antibiotics and illnesses at this stage, these can cause problems with hearing and balance. Your baby's taste buds are evident throughout her mouth and now connect to nerves, which will carry the taste sensation to the brain.	While most pregnancy symptoms have disappeared, you have not yet felt your baby move and you may wonder whether she is all right. This is normal, but try not to worry – rather enjoy the return of your old energy. A symptom that will become a reminder of your state of pregnancy is the emergence of 'preggy brain' – a foggy forgetfulness and disorganisation that worsens through pregnancy and lasts for a period after your baby arrives.
16	Watching your baby on an ultrasound, you may see her swallowing and notice movements of her facial muscles and lips. The brain tracts for facial muscles are functioning now, so your little one has facial expressions. Your baby may even suck her thumb and play with the umbilical cord. Studies have shown that more babies suck their right hand *in utero* and that the hand a baby sucks may indicate what her dominant hand will be. Your baby's eyes face forward and start moving in their sockets. She is about 11 cm long – around the size of a mango.	You may experience little aches and pains in your tummy and back. These are largely due to stretching of ligaments around your uterus. Your uterus now grows into the abdominal space. The upper part of the uterus (the *fundus*) will reach your belly button by week 20. The uterus pushes the intestines to the sides of the abdomen.

WEEK	Your baby's development	Your changing body
17	Now approximating the size of a banana, your baby is 13 cm long. Her skin is almost translucent and covered in a downy layer of hair called lanugo. While she gets all her oxygen through the umbilical cord, it occasionally looks like she is breathing. She is in fact practising breathing movements – preparing her lung and diaphragm muscles for taking her first breath. Your baby's skeleton is soft and still consists largely of cartilage, but will harden as the weeks go by. Practising body movements *in utero* is important not only for brain development but also for the formation of the muscles, joints and bones.	If this is your second or third pregnancy, you may feel your baby move around now but, for first-time moms, you will probably only feel your baby move between 20 and 22 weeks. At first it will feel like little flutters or butterflies in your tummy, or even gas bubbles but you will soon be able to identify your little baby's movements.
18	Your baby is around 14 cm now and is very active – kicking and moving to exercise those little muscles. The sex organs are well developed and if you are carrying a girl, her eggs are in place in her ovaries. Now is the time that the nerve tracts for touch and hearing develop, carrying sensations to the brain.	You may notice changes in bodily secretions, such as increased sweating. Vaginal discharge is common and nothing to worry about as long as it is clear – not bloody or smelly.

Things to do

- **Book a holiday**. If you are going to have a final holiday as a couple before your baby arrives, now is the time to book that trip. Travel between 22 and 32 weeks is best. You won't be able to fly late in your pregnancy so choose destinations that you can get to with ease in the next few months.
- **Investigate antenatal classes**. This is a good time to book antenatal classes. These are important as you prepare for delivering your baby. If you are empowered with knowledge your birth is more likely to go the way you wish.
- **Contact your medical scheme**. Register your pregnancy and clarify what cover you are eligible for.

Frequently asked questions

WHAT OVER-THE-COUNTER MEDICATION CAN I SAFELY TAKE IN PREGNANCY?

Approach any medication taken in pregnancy with caution. As a rule of thumb, ask your doctor or pharmacist. The following medication must **not** be taken in pregnancy:

- Aspirin and aspirin-containing products (e.g. Med-Lemon)
- Non steroidal anti-inflammatories (NSAIDS), including Voltaren, Ibuprofen and Nurofen, should not be taken, nor should combination painkillers such as Myprodol and Stopayne.

The following remedies are **safe** for common ailments:

Allergies and colds

- Lemsip is a safe option.
- Saline nasal sprays can be used for a blocked nose resulting from allergies or colds.
- Iliadin or Drixine nasal spray and drops (oxymetazoline) are useful for nasal congestion and safe in pregnancy. Do not use for longer than seven consecutive days.

Constipation

Movicol, Fybogel and Duphalac are safe treatments.

Gastro

- Fluid loss as a result of gastro-enteritis can be treated with Rehidrat or similar replacement solutions.
- Imodium can be used if necessary for diarrhoea.
- Probiotics are safe.

Heartburn

Rennie, Tums and Gaviscon can all be used for heartburn and indigestion.

Haemorrhoids

Piles can be treated with Preparation H, Poliherb, witch hazel and ice packs, Anusol ointment and suppositories.

Nausea

- Asic, two at night, one morning and lunchtime if necessary.
- Emex syrup 15–30 mℓ as required.

Pain and fever

Paracetamol (Panado) can be used in normal doses.

Vaginal candida (thrush)

Canesten (clotrimazole) can be used.

HINTS FOR THE OTHER HALF

- Your partner's body has changed significantly and she may need regular reassurance and affection. Touch her growing tummy – you will be able to feel the firm ball that is the uterus above the pubic bone.
- Look into the paternity leave allowance you have and apply for two weeks' leave around the due date of your baby.
- Is your home ready for the baby? Renovations always take longer and cost more than you anticipate, so don't leave this any longer than you have to.
- Is your car suitable for a baby? A two-door is less practical and harder on the back when dealing with car seats. Does your car have an isofix attachment belt for a baby seat to be secured?
- Give your partner focused attention at the end of each day. Switch off devices and prioritise uninterrupted time to talk about each other's day.
- If she needs a little TLC, run a bath or massage her back and feet.
- Read *Dad – The power and beauty of authentic fatherhood* by Craig Wilkinson. Your partner will appreciate your involvement.

The esSense of 14–18 weeks

- Moving into the second trimester brings a pleasant relief from nausea and fatigue. As you cannot feel your baby move yet, you may occasionally be concerned about your pregnancy and wonder if your baby is thriving.

- It is not necessary to have a scan at each appointment – your caregiver will get enough information from urine tests, blood pressure and an abdominal examination and measurement to confirm that everything is all right.

- You are gaining just over 1,5 kg a month and by the end of this stage you will probably have gained between 2,5 and 5 kg.

- Your baby is perfectly formed now and in this trimester many of the senses start to function. Although your baby cannot attach meaning to the sensory input, she begins to hear, smell and taste. She also looks like a perfect baby and even has facial expressions. She will grow to 14 cm by week 18.

CHAPTER 8

19–22 weeks

You have reached the halfway mark! Your pregnancy is flying by. Embrace this stage, which will be when you first feel your baby move, and is a pleasant month for most moms.

CARING FOR YOURSELF

Protein is very important in the second trimester. Protein-rich foods include egg, fish, meat, chicken, nuts and legumes such as lentils and chickpeas. Aim to include a palm-sized portion of protein at each mealtime. Healthy snacks are also helpful and a good habit to bridge the gap between meals. Snacks like nuts, seeds and low salt biltong are high in energy and proteins.

Supplements

A comprehensive antenatal supplement usually contains calcium, magnesium and vitamin D, all required for bone strength. If your diet is inadequate in these, a supplement is essential to prevent osteoporosis occurring in post-childbearing years.

Exercise

Continue to listen to your body as you maintain your exercise regimen of choice. Your changing body will tell you what exercise is safe and effective with your growing belly. It may be helpful to consult a personal fitness trainer or biokineticist to give you some guidelines for safe pregnancy exercise.

Weight gain

You will gain the most weight during this trimester (probably 1,6 kg per month) and by now it should be obvious that you are pregnant. Some first-time moms may still be able to hide their growing bump.

Making sense

Round ligament tendonitis is the term given to lower abdominal pain or tenderness, often experienced between weeks 16 and 26. The round ligaments are two ligaments on either side of the uterus that attach to the groin. As your uterus grows, they elongate and stretch, resulting in spasms, which frequently cause discomfort and pain. The pain is often one-sided (the uterus usually tilts more to one side), and is aggravated by movement, especially turning.

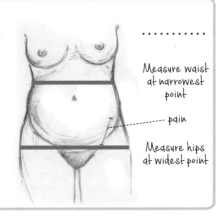

Measure waist at narrowest point

pain

Measure hips at widest point

Antenatal appointments

At your routine antenatal appointment your blood pressure and urine, and your baby's growth, will be measured. In addition, you will be referred for a detailed foetal anomaly scan, which is optimally performed between weeks 20 and 22.

In this scan, the size and structure of your baby and the placenta will be checked to detect any abnormalities. Ultrasound will be used to assess and measure the organs and body parts (heart, brain, spine, stomach, kidneys, bladder, genitalia, limbs).

In rare cases where problems are diagnosed, the knowledge is empowering:

- **Preparation** In the case of some anomalies, it is an enormous help to be prepared; for example, in the case of a cleft lip, you will be prepared for the appearance of your baby and have the opportunity to explore the successful outcomes of surgery and to prepare for feeding adjustments that might be necessary.
- **Pregnancy management** The findings might influence how the pregnancy is managed and where your baby should be born. For example, if your placenta is not functioning optimally, you may have more frequent antenatal visits or, in the case of a heart defect, may be advised to deliver at a hospital that has a neonatal ICU and a paediatric cardiologist on hand. In some cases, intrauterine therapies might be helpful, e.g. the drainage of excessive amniotic fluid.
- **Viability decision** Where appropriate, usually for a life-threatening abnormality or where quality of life is expected to be negligible, you may be offered the option of termination.

In view of the extremely sensitive outcome if anomalies are picked up, it is imperative that a skilled professional perform the anomaly scan. Foetal scanning has become a subspeciality, as skill and experience are important in picking up any abnormalities and also in being able to recognise what is normal.

> **MULTIPLE PREGNANCY**
>
> Hopefully the early nausea has lifted. You can eat the same amount of food as you would for a singleton pregnancy, but your level of exercise needs to be contained and monitored. You will gain more weight.
>
> Twin moms will usually require additional supplements. Iron deficiency anaemia is common, and an iron supplement and a multivitamin with **additional** calcium and vitamin D are recommended.
>
> As in singleton pregnancy, weight gain varies enormously. A recommended overall weight gain is 15,9 to 20,4 kg, or an average of 0,7 kg per week from 12 weeks.
>
> The 20–22 week anomaly scan is also recommended for twin pregnancy, as there is a slightly increased risk of congenital abnormalities with multiples.

BECOMING A MOM

Feeling your baby move will fill you with delight. Experiencing those little flutters and kicks and watching your baby on the ultrasound will help you start to bond. For some moms, bonding begins at conception and strengthens in this trimester as everything becomes more real. Others may be feeling detached and not fall in love yet. That's okay and does not mean that you will be a distant mom or battle to connect with your baby. For many moms bonding only starts after delivery – it's important to know that bonding and attachment is a journey that takes time.

During this trimester you will decide whether to find out your baby's gender now or at birth. If the baby is not the gender you wished for, you may be dealing with 'gender disappointment'. This is a complex emotion. You know that you should be feeling blessed, but you are disappointed and feel guilty for feeling this way. It will take time and support for you to come to terms with an altered dream. You may even experience this as a loss – the loss of a dream child – and have to pass through disbelief, despair and guilt before moving on to acceptance. The important thing is to know that you are not alone. Katherine Asbery, a psychologist who experienced this when she was expecting her third son, wrote a book that you might find helpful: *Altered Dreams – Living with gender disappointment.*

 Sensible pregnancy

When not to worry

Baby's size

Babies are individuals, and their sizes will vary. Don't worry if your baby measures bigger or smaller than average, as long as it is in the normal range and he is growing as expected.

A low-lying placenta

Placenta praevia, in which the placenta is attached low in the uterine cavity, covering all or part of the cervix, can only be diagnosed after 28 weeks. This is because the lower part of the uterus grows rapidly before this, and a placenta that is low early on, might be well clear of the cervix later.

If the placenta is reported as low at the 20-week scan, the position will be rechecked at 28 weeks. A low placenta at 20 weeks is not necessarily a *placenta praevia*. If the placenta is not covering the cervix at 20 weeks, it will probably not be low later.

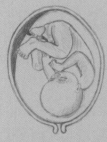 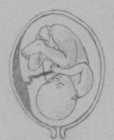 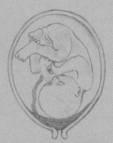

normal placenta   partial placenta previa   major placenta previa

Weekly progress

WEEK	Your baby's development	Your changing body
19	Your baby's skin starts to produce vernix, a white waxy coating. In time this will cover your baby's skin to protect it from the watery environment of the womb until birth and it may assist in a smoother slide down the birth canal. Your baby will sleep about 20 hours of each day, during which time you will still feel movement, but not as energetic as when he is awake. You may find your baby wakes up and moves more when you lie down to sleep at night – an indication that his vestibular system can now perceive movement and he uses the lulling motion of your movement to settle and sleep – just like a newborn does. He is 15,7 cm long.	As your baby starts to take up more space, you may find you occasionally experience heartburn and breathlessness. In first pregnancies you will start to feel movement in the next two weeks, and even earlier (around 17 weeks) in subsequent pregnancies. Although your baby moves vigorously, the first movements you become aware of will feel like flutters or bubbles.

WEEK	Your baby's development	Your changing body
20	The way we measure a baby's length changes at this point. Up to now we measured the foetus length from head to bum (16 cm this week), but now we will measure from head to heel (25 cm this week). As with every age-band norm, length varies between babies – they are individuals after all. Your baby swallows amniotic fluid that contains a few waste products and he produces urine now. Because he ingests waste products your baby starts to produce meconium – a sticky, dark green-black substance – in the bowel. This will be his first poo after birth and is made up of amniotic fluid, dead skin and hair cells and digestive secretions. 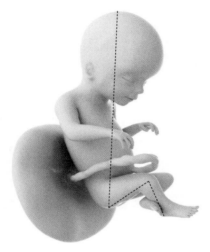	You are halfway through your pregnancy. Your uterus is pushing on your organs and your hormones have slowed down your digestion. This means that you may well have constipation at this point. The top (*fundus*) of the uterus is now at the level of your belly button. The uterus still feels like a ball or a melon – your caregiver cannot yet feel your baby's shape.
21	Your baby is now gaining weight rapidly, weighs around 350 g and is 27 cm long. He needs to lay down fat stores now in order to be ready to survive outside the womb. His eyelashes and eyebrows become evident at around this time.	Most of your weight gain will occur from 20 weeks on. You will probably gain about 400 g a week for the next 15 weeks, with the weight gain slowing down in the last month of pregnancy.
22	Your baby's senses are all fully functional – he can feel touch all over his body and finds comfort in sucking his thumb. He responds to sounds and can even track a light on your tummy with his eyes. Your baby has distinct eyebrows but his eye colour is not yet defined. His entire body is covered in lanugo – fine hair that some premature babies are born with – as well as vernix. There is meconium in his intestine that will not be released until your baby is born; in some babies this occurs during the birth process. Your little one is 28 cm long.	You are feeling your baby move more now. There is still enough space in the uterus for him to actively move and kick and you are aware of these movements.

Things to do

- **20-week scan** At your 20-week appointment you will be referred for a foetal anomaly scan to be done at 20 to 22 weeks to check for normality.
- **Focus on your diet** and giving your baby the best start. Choose foods high in iron, such as leafy dark veggies and red meat. Make sure you drink a lot of water to relieve constipation and eat foods rich in omegas.
- **Make your preferences known.** People will love to touch your expanding tummy and you may have strong feelings about this. If you don't want them doing this, let them know.

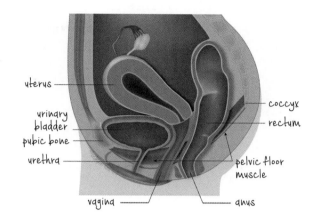

- **Pelvic floor exercises** It's time to start pelvic floor exercises (see p. 109). These are contractions of the muscles around the pelvic area that will be needed for the birth process as well as to prevent incontinence during and after pregnancy.

Frequently asked questions

CAN I TRAVEL IN PREGNANCY?

If you want to plan a holiday, the interval from weeks 20 to 32 is probably the best time. The exhaustion and nausea of early pregnancy will have passed, and you should not yet be experiencing the discomfort of late pregnancy.

Airlines will require a letter from your doctor after approximately 30 weeks (depending on the airline and whether a flight is domestic or international).

There is an increased risk of **thrombosis** (developing a clot) in pregnancy, but this risk is very low. Precautionary measures include increasing fluid intake, moving frequently, and wearing travel stockings.

Travel to **malaria areas** is not recommended in pregnancy. Pregnant women who develop malaria have an increased risk of complications and death, and there is no anti-malarial medication that is completely safe in pregnancy. Likewise it is not advisable to travel to countries with mosquitoes that carry the **Zika virus**. The Zika virus is transmitted by mosquitoes and linked to significant birth defects, specifically microcephaly (an abnormally small head) and brain abnormalities. The World Health Organization (WHO) has recommended that pregnant women do **not** travel to areas with active Zika virus transmission. If these areas are visited, measures must be taken to prevent mosquito bites, such as using mosquito repellents and covering up. These areas are Central and South America, the Caribbean, and the Pacific Islands.

It is sensible to avoid very **remote** destinations, extremely hot destinations and hectic itineraries! Also be sensible regarding activities – scuba diving and skiing are not recommended.

If your work requires travelling, plan ahead. Although you can travel on domestic flights a little later in pregnancy, if work involves flights early or late in the day, and long days of meetings, it would be wise to limit these trips after 30 weeks. Similar adjustments should be made if work involves long car trips.

When travelling:

- find out from your travel agent or airlines if a letter from your doctor is required;
- find out if any vaccinations are required, and if they are safe in pregnancy;
- know your blood group, your due date and an emergency contact for your obstetrician or midwife.

HINTS FOR THE OTHER HALF

- You are now halfway through 'your' pregnancy. Your partner will be starting to feel movements, but it's unlikely that you will be able to feel them yet.
- Attend the 20-week scan, as this is a detailed and important one, not to be missed. It is exciting to see your baby. If you don't want to know your baby's gender you will have to look away at certain moments, or the game will be given away!
- Research and book antenatal classes for you both. Your involvement in birth preparation classes is as important to you as to your partner. And you'll meet other couples and share your journey to parenthood (and realise you aren't alone dealing with a changed, sometimes unreasonable pregnant woman).
- Listen to your partner; hear her worries, as just sharing anxieties makes them manageable. Ask for details, explore ways to reduce her fears, let her know that her concerns matter to you, rather than minimising them. Share your thoughts, too, so she understands you, and can see your different perspective, which is no less important than hers.

The esSense of 19–22 weeks

- While your energy levels are high and this is generally a lovely part of pregnancy, you may experience some pregnancy niggles like heartburn, constipation and ligament pain.

- This month, you will have your detailed foetal anomaly scan, which looks at your baby's organs and growth, and also the health of the placenta. Because it informs many future decisions, it has to be done by someone with the required skills.

- You will be showing by now and your weight gain will increase to around 1,6 kg per month.

- Feeling your baby move brings a peace of mind to this stage of pregnancy.

- Your baby weighs around 350 g and, in the next half of pregnancy, the focus is your baby's growth and weight gain.

CHAPTER 9

23–27 weeks

This stage of pregnancy is generally a great period; you are not yet uncomfortably large and are still experiencing the energy of the second trimester. You are more than halfway there and, if your baby is born after 24 weeks, she has a strong chance of surviving outside the womb with medical assistance.

CARING FOR YOURSELF

Eat fresh, unprocessed and seasonal foods. You need only 340 g extra food and your diet should consist of three well-balanced meals made up of protein, three vegetables and a healthy carbohydrate. Include fresh fruit at least twice a day. Dairy products like unsweetened yoghurt, cheese and milk should be full cream.

Supplements

Continue to take your antenatal supplement. Your blood supply is increasing and new blood cells must be produced. For this reason, your body needs more iron than your dietary intake can meet. Some iron supplements should be taken an hour away from dairy foods for optimal absorption – read the instructions for your supplement.

Exercise

Your exercise regimen will have to adjust to meet the realities of your growing body, but don't be scared to continue what you can cope with. Make sure you drink sufficient fluids during and after exercise.

Weight gain

Your weight gain will continue at 1–2 kg a month and, if you are eating a healthy and unrefined diet, the weight gain should be well controlled.

Antenatal appointments

You are still having monthly antenatal appointments and during this phase of pregnancy, the routine checks discussed in Chapter 7 will be done at your antenatal visits:

- Urine tests for glucose, protein and signs of urinary tract infections
- Blood pressure
- Abdominal examination
- Ultrasound might be done.

MULTIPLE PREGNANCY

Ultrasound scans, at least once a month, are required to monitor the growth of twins; examining the abdomen is not accurate enough.

It takes longer to measure two babies than one, and you will need to get as comfortable as possible for the ultrasound scan. You may become breathless when you lie on your back so lie slightly towards one side during the scan.

It is unlikely that you will want or be able to work much beyond 32 or 34 weeks. Start planning for this now.

Pregnancy niggles

As your pregnancy progresses you will become more frustrated with little niggles related to your body changes. Always try to see these issues in the context of the miracle that is taking place in your body.

Leg cramps You may battle to sleep at night owing to restless legs or cramps in your calves. The exact cause of these symptoms isn't really understood, but there is often a significant improvement with a supplement of magnesium (Slow-Mag, Chela-Mag) taken at night. It is worth stretching your calf muscles before going to bed at night. If the calf cramps result in severe spasm, bending the knee and flexing the foot upwards can release it.

Shortness of breath Feeling short of breath with minimal exercise is very common now. The truth is that you are actually more efficient at oxygenation and shortness of breath is a perceived sensation by the brain. The growing uterus is pushing the diaphragm upwards and the ribcage splays outwards, adding to this sensation.

Palpitations Your heart beats approximately 10 beats per minute faster in pregnancy. You may have occasional runs of very rapid heartbeats, called supra-ventricular tachycardia (SVT). Although these can be normal, report them to your caregiver who will rule out anaemia, an overactive thyroid gland, and heart disease, which are other possible causes.

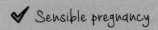
Food cravings

Almost every TV comedy featuring a pregnant woman will show her eating something strange like pickles with ice cream. While eating weird combinations of food or eating a lot of a certain type of food is common, pica is something entirely different. Pica is a condition of craving substances with little or no nutritional value. *Pica* is the Latin word for magpie, a bird notorious for eating almost anything. Most pica cravings involve non-food substances such as dirt or chalk.

Women suffering from pica commonly crave dirt, clay, and laundry starch. Other pica cravings include burnt matches, stones, charcoal, mothballs, ice, cornstarch, toothpaste, soap, sand, plaster, coffee grounds, bicarbonate of soda, and cigarette ashes.

If you start craving weird foods or non-food substances, don't panic; it happens and is not abnormal. Here are some suggestions to help you deal with pica cravings:
- Inform your caregiver to make sure you have a complete understanding of the specific risks associated with your cravings.
- Monitor your iron status along with your general vitamin and mineral intake.
- Consider potential substitutes for the cravings such as chewing sugarless gum.
- Ask a friend to help you avoid non-food items.

BECOMING A MOM

For most women, the second trimester is a time of calm and happiness – you are feeling better, have energy and are generally positive. The fatigue and nausea of the first trimester are a distant memory and the discomfort and exhaustion of the last trimester have not set in.

You may also experience mood swings and moments of ambivalence. One moment you feel happy and love your baby and the next you are anxious and not sure that this pregnancy was a good idea after all. This may go as far as feelings of resentment towards your unborn baby.

Rozsika Parker wrote about this 'maternal ambivalence' in her book *Torn in Two – The experience of maternal ambivalence*. She stresses the importance of recognising it as a normal process, saying that we need to accept that we will not always be the 'perfect mother' and may have distressing thoughts and feelings. In recognising this, we allow ourselves to be 'good enough' mothers. This awareness of not meeting the ideal frees us and 'contributes to the capacity to mother'.

This ambivalence is not uncommon; it just is not freely spoken about. You need to know that negative feelings are acceptable – they are part of the journey – and give yourself freedom to feel a range of positive and negative emotions. Try to manage these passing negative feelings by saying, "Right now I feel …". This helps you to keep the perspective that the emotion is transient and that tomorrow you could feel differently.

Weekly progress

WEEK	Your baby's development	Your changing body
23	Your baby is almost 29 cm long and weighs about 500 g. From now on it's a case of bulking up and laying down fat stores. As your baby fattens up, she will become less wrinkly too. Your baby's eyes are moving more and more – not yet in response to stimuli but certainly exercising those little extraocular muscles. The nerves carrying sound stimuli from the ear to the brain are becoming myelinated (covered with a coating that helps transmit the sensory impulse). This means that your little one will start to respond more to sounds over the upcoming weeks. Your baby hears your voice, the sound of your heartbeat and the gurgles of your digestive system. This white noise she hears *in utero* will be comforting to her after birth and is something you can use to help her sleep. Your baby's fingerprints are fully developed.	You may start to experience backache now that you are in the second half of pregnancy. Try to focus on good posture and get your feet up when you can.

WEEK	Your baby's development	Your changing body
24	For the first time, if born prematurely, your baby has a chance of survival (with help from technology). Her lungs start to produce surfactant between weeks 24 and 28. This is essential for breathing and survival after birth. Surfactant keeps the lungs inflated and prevents them from sticking together when your baby breathes out. Your baby's blood has been produced in the liver since 12 weeks. At around this time your baby's bone marrow starts to form blood cells. Now that your baby can hear, you may notice a startle reaction or jerk when she hears a loud and unexpected sound. Your baby is growing hair on her head, she is about 30 cm long – as long as a ruler – and weighs 630 g.	Your pregnancy affects every part of your body. Some women experience dry eyes and blurred vision in pregnancy. Others report nasal congestion and head cold symptoms. You may even have bleeding gums. Make notes of any concerns you have and ask your caregiver about them.
25	Your baby will be very active in the womb now, turning somersaults and kicking a lot. This movement is important for her muscle development. Her eyelids will open in the next week and she is starting to respond to light. If a light is shone on your tummy, your baby may turn towards it and even track the light if it is moved across the tummy. Your baby starts to bed down fat layers, which are vital for warmth and energy after she is born. She weighs around 676 g and is 33 cm long.	You are approaching the end of your second trimester so enjoy the last few weeks of feeling energised. In the third trimester you will find yourself getting more tired and needing to rest more frequently. The uterus has now grown further into the abdominal cavity, reaching well beyond the level of your belly button. The wall of the uterus is thinner, and your baby's body parts can be felt – it might be possible to determine how she is lying. Your baby's movements are more obvious.
26	All parts of your baby's eyes are formed. Her eyelids have been closed until now, even though she could see, but at around this time she will open her eyes and soon start to blink. Your baby starts to perceive, integrate and learn from sounds and will react to familiar sounds like your voice. She is now around 35 cm long and has about another 15 cm to grow before birth. She has fingernails.	Braxton Hicks contractions (see p. 87) start. These are irregular tightening of the uterine muscles, not strong or coordinated enough to result in dilatation of the cervix. They are not the contractions of labour. You may be quite unaware of these contractions, especially in your first pregnancy.

WEEK	Your baby's development	Your changing body
27	Your baby weighs about 880 g and is 37 cm. If born now, there is a strong likelihood that she will survive with special care. The last stage of pregnancy is vital and focuses on growth, brain development and lung maturity. Your baby's sense of touch begins to carry tactile input to the part of the brain designated for touch (the somatosensory cortex). She will feel touch input consciously for the first time. This means that from now on your baby can feel pain. Your baby is active about 10–30 per cent of the time.	Your appetite starts to increase and you may crave foods that you don't really need, like sugary snacks. Try to watch your intake carefully and eat healthy, nutritious food, not empty calories. Your body will begin to produce colostrum – an early form of milk (see p. 18). Some women occasionally leak this discharge from their breasts from around now to the end of pregnancy.

Things to do

- **Monitor your mood**. If you are feeling down and apprehensive about becoming a mother, talk to your partner or mom and, if necessary, seek the support of a counsellor or psychologist. This will help you prepare for your new role.
- **Take antenatal classes**. If you haven't started antenatal classes, now is the time. These classes will give you information about pregnancy, labour and parenting a newborn baby, and also provide an opportunity to network with other expectant parents. If you want a natural delivery these classes are essential, as a good antenatal class will teach you about the signs of labour and how to breathe through each stage of labour. A childbirth educator or midwife usually gives these classes. The style of the classes, as well as the content, will vary tremendously. Take a little time to find out what will suit you. Speaking to friends and acquaintances who have attended antenatal classes will give you insight, as will a phone call or a visit to a website. Some parents might prefer not to attend antenatal classes, or might prefer an online course, or a one-on-one session with a midwife.
- **Plan the nursery**. You can start to plan your baby's nursery now and make a list of what you need to buy (see Chapter 13, p. 114). Bear in mind that having a baby is expensive, so try to prioritise pre-baby purchases – some may not really be necessary.
- **Create a birth plan**. It's time to starting thinking about your birth preferences. At this stage, it is too early to finalise it, as so much can still change. Your antenatal classes and Chapters 13-16 will guide you. Later on you might want to write something down to share and discuss with your caregiver.

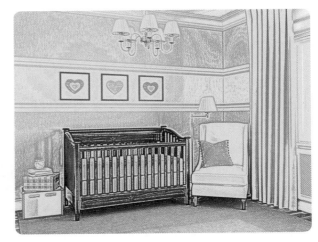

Frequently asked questions

CAN I LIE ON MY BACK?

The *vena cava* is a large, thin-walled vein that returns blood to the heart, and lies behind the uterus. Once the uterus is large enough, it might compress this vein when you lie flat on your back. This results in a temporary decrease in the blood returning to the heart, and a drop in blood pressure (Supine Hypotensive Syndrome), resulting in dizziness, nausea and sweating in the mom. This can lead to a drop in your baby's heart rate. These changes all resolve when you turn on your side.

For this reason it is sensible to avoid lying flat on your back. As long as the upper part of the body is elevated (propped up by pillows), or you lie slightly to one side (either side), this can be avoided. But if you wake up lying on your back, don't worry: your baby is fine; just shift position to your side.

HINTS FOR THE OTHER HALF

- Plan together, initiating conversations about the baby, your hopes and dreams for her and your family and parenting roles. Talk about how the family you grew up in worked or didn't work, what you'd like to do similarly, what you'd like to do differently. What rituals and religious aspects are important to you?
- Enthusiastically attend childbirth preparation classes. Apart from the importance of showing your love and commitment to your partner, attending classes makes your impending fatherhood that much more real, enabling you to understand things better and feel more confident.
- You will feel your baby moving in your partner's tummy and can even play games with her, gently pushing poky bits, and responding when they poke out again … your first hide-and-seek!
- Your baby can hear your voice and becomes familiar with it, even recognising you when she is born, so it is a good idea to talk in her presence as much as possible.
- Show financial responsibility in your planning and spending, and discuss finances, particularly if your joint income will be less once your baby arrives. Budgets can be discussed and implemented in anticipation.

The esSense of 23–27 weeks

- While the second trimester glow continues, you may start to experience shortness of breath, heart palpitations and leg cramps.

- You will still be gaining over a kilogram a month.

- Your baby is around 35 cm long and has another 15 cm to grow before birth. Much of what happens now is growth related, rather than the formation of new structures.

- By 24 weeks, your baby can hear. Over the next few months she will respond to noise and in the third trimester he starts to recognise your voice.

- Your check-ups continue to be monthly and the routine checks of urine and blood pressure, and abdominal examination are par for the course.

CHAPTER 10

28–32 weeks

As you go into your third trimester, your mind turns with anticipation to your baby's birth. If your baby is born now, he will have a good chance of survival with the help of modern technology.

CARING FOR YOURSELF

You are now in your third trimester. Your uterus and your baby have grown extensively and you will notice that your capacity for large meals decreases as your digestive organs get pushed aside for the growing baby. This may necessitate smaller meals and more substantial snacks. You can ensure adequate calorie intake with less volume by including some healthy fats like avocados, olives, nuts and seeds and coconut oil. The benefit of including these fats is that you are more likely to meet your growing baby's essential fatty acid demands, which are critical for brain and eye development.

Supplements

It is a good idea to add omega 3 to your antenatal supplement during this trimester. The focus in this trimester is laying down neural pathways in your growing baby's brain, hence the increased demand for omega 3.

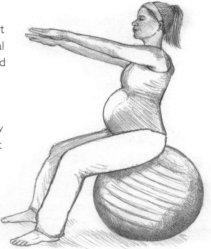

Exercise

You may need to adjust or change your exercise regime to safely accommodate your growing belly. It is important to be active, but don't overdo it.

Weight gain

You will continue to gain weight during this time but may notice it slows down a bit. As long as your doctor is happy with your and your growing baby's health, don't fret about what the scale says.

Constipation

If you suffer from constipation, you are in good company. It frequently occurs in the final months of pregnancy. Constipation is common in pregnancy owing to:
• hormone changes that slow down digestion; and
• iron supplements, which can exacerbate constipation.

Manage constipation during pregnancy as follows:
• Eat regularly. Small, frequent meals can help prevent constipation.
• Drink plenty of fluids, especially water; aim for 8–10 glasses a day.

- Exercise every day. Simple activities, such as daily walks, can be effective.
- Eat high-fibre foods, such as fruit, vegetables and legumes.
- Stool softeners (e.g. Movicol, Laxette) add moisture to the stool, making it easier to pass, and are safe to take in any trimester in pregnancy. The body doesn't absorb the active ingredients in these products, so they're unlikely to have an effect on the foetus.

Don't take any other type of laxative without first discussing it with your doctor.

Antenatal appointments

Your caregiver will see you every three to four weeks now. At these appointments your caregiver will check your urine and blood pressure, examine your abdomen to assess your baby's growth and the amniotic fluid, and address any concerns you may have about your current symptoms.

LOW-LYING PLACENTA

If your placenta was found to be low-lying at the 20-week scan, a repeat ultrasound is due now to see if it remains low (see *placenta praevia*, p. 75).

Blood tests

ANAEMIA

Anaemia (low red blood cell count) in pregnancy is common and is usually the result of iron deficiency. If you are feeling tired and short of breath, you may have anaemia. It can also aggravate headaches and heart palpitations.

Whether or not you have signs of anaemia, your haemoglobin level will probably be checked at this time. If you do have anaemia, there may be further investigation to determine its cause – iron, vitamin B12, folate, or other deficiency or another cause. It is usually treated with appropriate supplements.

RHESUS ANTIBODIES

If your blood type is rhesus negative (Rh–), a repeat blood test should be done for antibodies. The first test for antibodies would have been done at the beginning of the pregnancy.

If you are rhesus negative and have been exposed to rhesus positive (Rh+) blood from a blood transfusion or a previous pregnancy, your body will form antibodies to the rhesus factor. These antibodies can cross the placenta and cause anaemia or other serious complications in rhesus positive babies. For this reason, if your blood group is negative, you will be tested for antibodies earlier in pregnancy and again at 28 and 36 weeks of pregnancy. You won't know your baby's blood group until he is born, unless both his dad and you are rhesus negative, in which case he will be negative.

If you are Rh– a sample of blood will be taken from the umbilical cord at birth to test your baby's blood group. If he is Rh+, you will be given an anti-D injection that will prevent the development of antibodies. This is essential to prevent complications with subsequent pregnancies.

> **MULTIPLE PREGNANCY**
>
> You will have two antenatal visits in this period. This increased monitoring is because of the increased risk of preeclampsia, premature labour and placental problems with twin pregnancy.
>
> It is also time to start researching practical aspects – including car seats that will fit your car and twin prams. Groups such as SAMBA (the South African Multiple Birth Association) provide practical and emotional support.

> **Making sense**
> . . . .
>
> Major *placenta praevia* describes a placenta that covers the cervix. Vaginal birth is not possible, and there is an associated risk of significant bleeding.

Some doctors recommend routinely giving an anti-D injection to all Rh− mothers at 28 weeks of pregnancy to prevent any possible formation of antibodies.

Discuss these options with your obstetrician or midwife.

Pregnancy niggles

HEARTBURN AND REFLUX

Indigestion results in unpleasant symptoms that can occur at any stage in pregnancy, but frequently in the third trimester. They include heartburn, reflux, heaviness in the centre of the chest, bloating, nausea and vomiting, and even coughing.

The hormone changes of pregnancy relax muscles and allow the acidic contents of the stomach to move back up the oesophagus. This is exacerbated as pregnancy progresses and the increasingly bigger uterus pushes up against the stomach.

To manage heartburn, eat smaller meals, avoid eating shortly before going to bed, avoid lying flat and avoid foods that aggravate it (often pastry, bread). Medication is frequently required — antacids or acid suppressants (e.g. Gaviscon, Rennies, or any brand of ranitidine or omeprazole).

Severe heartburn or pain under your ribs might be a warning sign of preeclampsia and needs to be checked. It is a myth that heartburn occurs because your baby has lots of hair.

VARICOSE VEINS AND HAEMORRHOIDS

These are two more unpleasant side effects of pregnancy. The hormones progesterone and relaxin cause blood vessels to dilate, and the increasing size of the uterus puts pressure on the veins of the legs, genitalia and around the anus.

Varicose veins are dilated veins, usually in the legs but sometimes also in the groin and vulva. They can be large and bendy or small and spider-like. They are unattractive and can be uncomfortable but don't usually cause serious problems. They improve dramatically after delivery, although they don't disappear completely. There will be a temporary improvement with elevation of the legs. Graduated elastic stockings can also provide relief; these should be individually fitted to prevent overly tight stockings from making the veins worse.

Piles or haemorrhoids are varicose veins around the anus. They can be internal, within the anal canal, or external, protruding out of the anus. They cause discomfort, itching and pain, and frequently bleed. The bleeding is bright red blood, noticed either in the toilet bowl or on wiping after passing a stool. Piles are managed using topical ointments or suppositories to reduce the inflammation (e.g. Anusol or Scheriproct) and stool softeners if they are aggravated by constipation. Piles rarely require surgery during pregnancy.

Although they often get worse with delivery, haemorrhoids improve significantly after a few weeks, usually disappearing completely.

BECOMING A MOM

As your journey towards motherhood gathers speed, you may feel unsettled by the loss of the woman you were. You may feel more dependent and need help at times, making you feel vulnerable. You may also be treated differently – as if you are fragile. For an emancipated woman who has been in charge of her own life, this feeling can create turmoil.

Weekly progress

WEEK	Your baby's development	Your changing body

28	Your baby is about 38 cm long and now weighs over a kilogram.
	    The third trimester is a stage of rapid brain growth and over the next few weeks your baby's brain will start to control some bodily functions. His brain already controls reflexive and breathing movements, and coordinates sucking and swallowing. Heart rate, blood pressure and breathing are also under the control of his brain, which is why 90 per cent of babies born from this time on can survive with support. Temperature regulation, which is needed for survival, is not developed yet.
	    Eyebrows, eyelids and eyelashes are all visible and your baby opens and closes his eyes. Vision develops from now onwards through pregnancy. It is the least developed sense at birth and your baby will only be able to focus 20 cm away – exactly right to see your eyes while he is at the breast.
		In the last trimester of pregnancy you will be needing to wee more and may also experience constipation. Your baby's body parts and the way he is lying can be easily felt. His movements are more vigorous and other people can feel them too.

29	At 1,1 kg your baby weighs a third of his birth weight and is 39 cm long. From now on growth is the name of the game.
	    If you are having a boy, his testicles will descend through the groin as they head towards the scrotum. Your little girl has all her reproductive organs and eggs in place and her clitoris is large and visible, as it's not yet covered by the labia.
	    Your baby's sense of taste is functioning now and he shows strong preferences for sweet tastes by swallowing more frequently when you eat sweet foods.
		You may experience swelling of your legs and feet, especially if you stand for too long. In addition, varicose veins may plague your last stage of pregnancy.

WEEK	Your baby's development	Your changing body
30	In the next few weeks, space in the uterus will decrease but your little one needs to use the space that still exists to turn into the head-down position, ready for birth. The vestibular system in the inner ear senses gravity and will play a role in your baby's turning head down. He weighs about 1,3 kg and is now 40 cm long. He will grow about 10 cm in the next 10 weeks.	You may be aware of Braxton Hicks contractions, although some mothers don't experience them until the last few weeks of pregnancy. You will probably become aware of your baby having the hiccups. He will do so frequently and it is surmised that hiccups develop the lungs, exercising the diaphragm ready for breathing. Once you've recognised this rhythmic movement, there's no missing it.
31	Your baby's fingers are perfectly formed, his fingernails are growing and he can even scratch himself. Each finger has its unique fingerprint – your baby's identity for life. His bones are still soft but start to harden up in the third trimester, which means his need for calcium is high and you need to ensure you are eating plenty of calcium-rich foods. By the seventh month of pregnancy your baby's brain has developed every brain cell he will have for life. From now onwards the brain's role is to make connections (synapses) between the cells to make sense of the world. The cortical (thinking and control) part of your baby's brain starts to function and in the last 12 weeks of pregnancy your baby learns things such as recognising certain sounds (your voice) and the memory of a stimulus. He is 41 cm long.	From now on your weight gain will slow down, while your baby's increases as he still needs to fatten up considerably before 40 weeks. You will start to feel tired and breathless at times. Respect your amazing body by setting aside time to rest every day.
32	Your baby starts to behave like a newborn, playing and moving, practising newborn movements when awake. At this stage, he has a 95 per cent chance of survival if born prematurely. Your baby still sleeps 90 per cent of every day and is developing his sleep cycles. He also starts to move his eyes rapidly during REM (rapid eye movement) sleep and appears to be dreaming. In the last two months of pregnancy your baby starts losing the downy layer of hair (lanugo) that covers him. These hairs are swallowed along with the amniotic fluid and will be part of what makes up your baby's meconium – his dark, sticky, tar-like first poo. Measuring 43 cm and weighing 1,7 kg, your little one is plumping up nicely in preparation to thrive after birth. He will need some extra fat stores at birth as all babies lose a bit of weight in the days after birth.	Insomnia sets in as you become more uncomfortable. This adds to the fatigue of carrying a lot of extra weight and you will be tired and a little emotional.

Things to do

- **Start turning your mind to birth**. It is time to read Chapter 13 of this book – In preparation (see p. 107). This chapter will guide your preparation for birth over the next 10 weeks.
- **Talk to your baby**. Now that your baby can hear and starts to recognise your home language, talk to him – this will enhance his recognition of you after birth
- **Avoid sleeping on your back**. Now that your uterus and baby are heavier, you should avoid sleeping on your back to prevent the weight of the uterus from pressing on the vein that returns blood to the heart, dropping your blood pressure. This isn't good for your baby and may make you feel nauseous and faint. You will be more comfortable on your side.
- **Pack a hospital bag**. Pack reading material, maternity pads, a comfortable feeding bra, pyjamas and toiletries including lip balm (see p. 110 for a full list).
- **Take a hospital tour**. As you prepare for birth, now is the time to take a tour of the hospital. It is also worth finding a lactation consultant and getting your head around breast-feeding – it doesn't always come naturally.

Frequently asked questions

MY DUE DATE KEEPS CHANGING – WHEN IS MY BABY DUE?

The calculated due date is an estimation only. It is based on the first day of the last menstrual period with an estimate of when you ovulated and conceived.

An ultrasound scan done before 16 weeks of pregnancy, based on the foetus size, is very accurate in dating the pregnancy. If the scan is in agreement with the calculated date (to within five days), the latter date is taken as correct. Otherwise, the ultrasound date is used.

Later ultrasounds measure your baby's size and relate it to the average baby. For example, if you are 30 weeks pregnant but your baby is larger than average, you might be told that your baby measures the same size as the average 32-week-old baby. This doesn't mean that you are now 32 weeks pregnant or that your baby will come two weeks earlier. It merely means that he is bigger than average.

Pregnancy is humbling in that such an exceptionally important event cannot be predicted exactly, even with all the smart technology available!

HINTS FOR THE OTHER HALF

- Your baby is viable, so could survive if born now.
- Show your appreciation and enjoyment of your partner's changing body, and think of ways to make her feel special. *The 5 Love Languages* by Gary Chapman is a great book to read and implement at this time.
- Apply for two to three weeks' paternity leave if you can. Two days is not nearly long enough. You will want to prioritise spending a chunk of time at home getting to know your baby, helping Mom and becoming a competent, involved dad right from the get-go.
- Conflict is an unavoidable part of relationships and needs to be dealt with well. If you have destructive ways of dealing with conflict, now is the best time to have a few couples counselling sessions. Once the baby arrives you will be emotionally and physically much more distracted and busy. The journey to parenthood is full of mistakes and imperfections, and you both need to be accomplished at apologising to each other and fighting fair.
- Discuss any away trips from now until the birth, as you don't want to risk not being around when it happens. Your partner may find travelling tough from now on, and air travel may be restricted.

The esSense of 28–32 weeks

* Your regular visits to your caregiver involve the usual checks and may include testing for anaemia. If your blood group is negative, you will also have a rhesus antibody test.

* By the end of this stage, you may start to have more frequent check-ups.

* Your uterus pushes up on the stomach and this means that stomach contents may be regurgitated due to lax muscles at the top of the tummy. This causes heartburn and reflux, which you can treat with safe over-the-counter medication.

* You may be able to feel your baby's body parts through your tummy and may notice regular little hiccups. You may also start to feel the tightening contractions that are Braxton Hicks – they are not pre-labour warning signs, just your uterine muscles exercising.

* Your baby's weight is one third of what it will be at birth and he still has a lot of fattening up to do. You, on the other hand, will gain less weight in the last trimester than you did in the second.

CHAPTER 11

33–37 weeks

You are into the home stretch. If your baby is born in this period she may not even need technology to ensure her survival. Twins are usually delivered towards the end of this month.

CARING FOR YOURSELF

Continue to follow a well-balanced diet with lots of vegetables and fresh fruits, low in refined carbs (sugar, baked goods, pasta and breads). Protein intake is critical to maintain the health of the placenta. You can increase your protein intake by including a daily protein shake or two eggs a day over and above your dairy and meat proteins.

Supplements

Don't cut back on your supplements. You are feeding your baby and also need to replenish your own stores, so they remain important.

Exercise

You may need to taper off the intensity of exercise, as you may tire more rapidly around this stage. Just some gentle walks are enough to keep your lungs and heart healthy. In preparation for birth your body is producing a hormone called relaxin, which allows your pelvic ligaments to relax. As a result you may experience pelvic pain while walking. Be careful of overstretching.

Weight gain

Your weight gain usually slows down significantly and you may experience a small amount of weight loss leading up to birth. Again, if you and baby are healthy, don't sweat the numbers.

Heartburn and diet

You may find that your growing baby puts pressure on your digestive tract, forcing stomach contents back up through the oesophagus. You can minimise acid reflux or heartburn by eating small, regular meals, chewing food thoroughly and eating slowly. Don't lie down for at least an hour after eating.

To minimise symptoms of heartburn try to avoid:
- too many refined starches like cakes and white bread;
- spicy foods like curries and chilli sauces;
- rich, creamy foods like cream sauces and gravies;
- overeating at any meal, no matter what the food is.

Baby's position

It's getting tight in there but there is still enough room to move and your baby will shift the position of her back from one side to the other. In this period she will probably be in a head-down (vertex) position.

It is not yet a concern if your baby is not lying head down. Only 3 to 4 per cent of babies will be breech (head up towards your ribs) by full term. No intervention is necessary before 37 weeks of pregnancy.

If your baby is still breech at 37 weeks, your caregiver will discuss options with you. Very few obstetricians or midwives will offer vaginal birth as an option if your baby is breech, as this position does create higher risk of death for your baby if delivered vaginally. C-section reduces the risks to the baby in labour and results in a better outcome for newborns.

If there are no contraindications (such as high blood pressure, previous C-section or poor foetal growth), the option of turning your baby, known as external cephalic version (ECV), may be discussed. This reduces the need for a C-section and is rarely associated with complications.

ECV involves pushing on your abdomen and attempting to turn the baby in a somersault-like motion. This should be accompanied by monitoring before and afterwards and is usually done in a labour ward. ECV is successful in approximately 50 per cent of cases.

There are alternative options for turning your baby, such as reflexology, postural management, chiropractic and acupuncture. While there is no scientific evidence that these methods are effective, if you have time before your C-section is being scheduled, you may explore these options.

> **MULTIPLE PREGNANCY**
>
> You will have an antenatal visit at least every two weeks.
>
> For twins who share a placenta, delivery is advised at 36 completed weeks. If each twin has her own placenta, delivery at 37 weeks is recommended. Continuing pregnancy beyond 38 weeks increases the risk of foetal death in twin pregnancies.
>
> C-section delivery is usually recommended for twins. There is evidence of increased risk to the second twin with vaginal birth. If your preference is for vaginal birth, this may be considered if the first twin is head down and there are no other complications.

Antenatal appointments

For the last month before your baby arrives, you will probably be seeing your doctor or midwife weekly.

SWAB TEST

You may be offered a screening test for Group B Streptococcus (GBS) at 37 weeks of pregnancy. GBS bacteria are normally found in the vagina in 10 to 30 per cent of women, not causing any infection. If GBS is detected, there is a small chance that it can be transmitted to your baby during labour, possibly causing a serious infection in your newborn.

Some advice recommends testing all pregnant women in late pregnancy by taking a swab (with a cotton bud) from the vagina and rectum. If the swab tests positive, you will receive treatment with intravenous antibiotics in labour to reduce the risk of infection.

Pregnancy niggles

For many women, particularly in the first pregnancy, this remains an easy stage of pregnancy, although discomfort does start to increase towards 37 weeks. For others the physical burden of pregnancy becomes quite uncomfortable. Keep in mind that it is temporary and the result will be well worth it.

ACHES AND PAINS

You are possibly experiencing upper and lower backache, pain over the symphysis pubis (the central joint between the pubic bones), and pain from the sacroiliac joint (the joint between the sacrum and the iliac bones at the back of the pelvis, fairly central to each buttock). These niggles are the side effects of hormones and weight gain:

- Progesterone and relaxin soften your ligaments significantly, causing an increase of movement in the joints.
- The weight and size of the uterus and its contents, as well as the increasing weight of your breasts, put new strains on your body and change your centre of gravity.

It is often a matter of trial and error to find what will help most:

- Light exercise and keeping moving do help. Water-based exercise is probably the most comfortable.
- Massage and physiotherapy can be beneficial.
- Elasticated pregnancy support belts that provide support for the pelvis and lower abdomen help relieve symptoms.

A common complaint is a stitch-like pain under one or both ribs. This is probably as a result of pressure on the phrenic nerve, which supplies the diaphragm. Changing position and sitting more upright usually brings a little relief.

Pelvic girdle pain (which includes symphysis pubis dysfunction or SPD) affects one in five pregnancies. There is a range, from normal pain to women who are quite severely affected (see p. 95).

Sleeping is frequently disrupted by the need to get up and pass urine, and the discomfort experienced when turning in bed. A pillow to support your belly and a pillow between the legs are helpful.

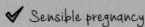

✔ Sensible pregnancy

When to call your caregiver

Your need to call your midwife or doctor if you experience any of the following:

Bleeding

In general bleeding in pregnancy is considered abnormal. A small amount of bleeding can occur after intercourse or if there is inflammation due to a vaginal infection, such as candida (thrush). However, if you are bleeding more than this, or if it is accompanied by pain, you need to seek medical attention immediately.

Warning signs of preeclampsia

Preeclampsia is a serious disorder of pregnancy, which is diagnosed by raised blood pressure and/or the presence of protein in the urine. If you experience a severe headache, changes in vision (either blurred vision or flashing lights), severe pain in the upper abdomen or below the ribs, vomiting in the third trimester, or a sudden onset of swelling of the face, hands or feet, you need to have your blood pressure and urine checked the same day.

Labour

Labour before 37 completed weeks is premature and your baby needs to be assessed to ensure she is fine to determine whether it is appropriate to attempt to stop labour. The mucous plug ('sign' or 'show') may precede the onset of contractions. This is usually a slimy, mucus-like discharge mixed or streaked with blood. Regular painful contractions, leakage or gush of amniotic fluid, passing the mucous plug, or *any* bleeding are signs that must be reported immediately.

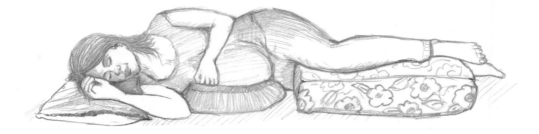

SWELLING

Swelling (oedema) occurs because the normal changes of pregnancy allow fluid to 'leak' out of the small capillaries into the tissues. It tends to be gravity driven, affecting feet and legs, hands, the lower abdomen and the vulva. Swelling increases later in pregnancy and is worse when the weather is hot and humid. Swelling will disappear within the first week of delivery.

If there is a sudden and dramatic onset of swelling, have it checked out. Women who develop preeclampsia (a complication characterised by high blood pressure and protein in the urine) usually have marked swelling.

Compressed nerves due to swelling in the tissues of the wrist may result in pain, tingling, numbness and clumsiness, often affecting some fingers more than others. This is Carpal Tunnel Syndrome and sometimes needs attention. It gets worse when the hands are still, and improves with movement. Try to elevate your hands and wrists at night or get a wrist splint. Your doctor may prescribe a high dose of vitamin B (Neurobion).

> MAKING SENSE
>
> **Pelvic girdle pain** (PGP) or pubic symphysis pain (PSP) refers to excessive pelvic instability and pain in the pelvis, lower back, lower abdomen and legs, and is due to the laxity of the supporting ligaments, and increased movement of the joints of the pelvis.
>
> Management is difficult, usually a combination of pain killers, pelvic support devices, avoidance of aggravating movements and, if necessary, crutches.

Baby's movements

Your baby takes up more space in your abdomen now, pushing up against the diaphragm and pushing your intestines further to the sides. There will always be enough space for her. She is surrounded by amniotic fluid to move around in and will be more flexed, with her legs drawn up against her body.

Movement is a reassuring sign of your baby's wellbeing and you will become familiar with its pattern. There will be quiet times when she sleeps and busier times, often after you have eaten or when you are lying down. Strong kicks can be felt but, as she grows, the movement you feel is more frequently due to rolling and stretching. The number of movements felt increases until 32 weeks, then remains much the same.

The movements continue, but are more squirming than brisk kicks. Be aware of your baby's movements in general, although it is not necessary to actually count or monitor them.

If you are concerned that there is less movement than usual, lie on your left side and count the movements over two hours – you should feel 10 or more definite movements. Take some deep breaths and drink something sweet. If movement is indeed reduced, report this to your caregiver on the same day.

BECOMING A MOM

You will be feeling quite ready to give birth. The physical discomfort towards the end of this final stage will mean that you are preoccupied with how to get the labour process started and feel a sense of urgency to deliver a healthy baby.

If you have an extreme fear of delivery (see tokophobia, p. 33), make your caregiver aware of your fear. Discuss the basis of the fear and whether planning a more predictable delivery – possibly a C-section – may ease your fears.

Weekly progress

WEEK	Your baby's development	Your changing body
33	Your baby weighs around 1,9 kg and is 44 cm long. She will turn head down soon and her bones are becoming harder. Her skull bones will not fuse yet and remain flexible for the squeeze through the birth canal and to allow for brain growth after birth. Sensory input – sounds, tastes and smells in particular – that your baby is exposed to *in utero* will be the ones she prefers after birth. We know that babies who taste strongly flavoured foods, such as liquorice, curry and chilli, accept more varied tastes later and we suspect that a varied diet in pregnancy will lead to less fussy eating in the toddler years. After birth, your baby will recognise and show preference for your voice and the language you speak.	Your mind will be preoccupied with the birth at this stage. This preoccupation with your baby's safety and life will remain for a long time after the birth.
34	At 45 cm and 2,1 kg, your baby is running out of space *in utero* and her movements slow down a little as she becomes more cramped. You will still feel movement right to the end and possibly including regular little jerks which are an indication that your baby has hiccups. As your baby moves against resistance and touches her body, she starts to develop a sense of 'me' versus 'not me' that will be refined significantly in the first six months after birth As your baby grows, the uterine and belly walls stretch and get thinner so more light gets through to your baby. She will watch for light and respond by tracking lights and shadows when awake. If your baby is a boy, his testes will now reach his scrotum and his genitals will look like those of a full-term baby boy.	A certain amount of swelling in your hands, feet and legs is normal and you will have noticed it increasing in the last few weeks. If you have a sudden increase in swelling, especially if it is accompanied by headaches or changes in vision, have this checked – it may be a sign of preeclampsia.
35	Your baby is over 46 cm and weighs around 2,3 kg. From now until term, she will gain almost 230 g per week, fattening out nicely. She has a strong grasp and is ready to hold your finger when she is born. Your baby continues to shed the lanugo, the hair that has covered her body for much of the pregnancy. She swallows this hair along with the amniotic fluid and the liver and kidneys are becoming capable of processing waste.	At around this time, you may feel the relief of breathing easier, as your baby drops down into your pelvis, getting ready for birth.
36	By eight months, each brain cell is perfectly formed, has migrated to its place within the brain and is making connections and, in doing so, provides the platform for learning and physical development. Your baby has double the number of brain cells of an adult brain and there is a confusing mesh of networks that are largely unnecessary. The brain now enters a time of pruning – getting rid of brain cells that are ineffective or not useful. Brain cells that are in the right place and useful are used and networks are reinforced, but others are lost – it's literally a case of 'Use it or lose it'. This pruning takes place throughout life but is dramatic in childhood. Your baby now measures 48 cm and weighs around 2,6 kg.	You are into the final month of pregnancy and will be feeling ready to have your baby – in fact, perhaps desperate for her to be born. Your pelvic joints will loosen even further, which may cause extreme discomfort when you walk.

WEEK	Your baby's development	Your changing body
37	While your baby is considered full-term now and is ready to be born, the next two weeks are still important for fattening up and some lung development. She will weigh around 2,8kg and is 49 cm long. Your baby is curled up tightly as there is not a lot of space in the womb. She will be in this curled up position for the first two weeks after birth – we call it physiological flexion and her first movement task after birth will be to stretch out and develop her back muscles.	It's time to start watching for early labour signs that include a show (a mucous substance in your panties with a streak of blood), your waters breaking or contractions like very strong Braxton Hicks that you can't breathe through with ease.

Things to do

- **Arrange a photoshoot**. You are still glowing and your tummy is gorgeous. Fit in a shoot now, before you become too bloated and puffy with water retention prior to the birth of your baby.
- **Prepare your pantry**. It's time to stock up the kitchen and freezer with easy-to-prepare meals and nutritious snacks for after you come home from the hospital.
- **Pack your hospital bag**. It's time to pack your baby's hospital bag. She will need newborn clothes, nappies and a swaddling blanket.
- **Practise perineal massage**. From 37 weeks perineal massage may increase the flexibility of the opening to the vagina and gets you familiar with your perineal anatomy (see Chaper 13).
- **Prepare your birth plan**. It is time to start preparing your birth plan. Download examples of birth plans and chat to your partner about preferences such as where to give birth, pain relief, how your baby will be delivered and what you want to happen right after birth.

Frequently asked questions

How long should I continue working?

Although many mothers feel they would like to work as long as possible, saving most of their maternity leave for after the birth, it is recommend that you stop work at least two weeks before your due date. Towards the end of pregnancy you will be more uncomfortable and probably feel less driven and interested in work. Having some time to 'nest' and get organised for your baby, as well as time to relax and rest, is good for you and therefore good for your baby. In the weeks to come, you will probably be grateful you took this time.

Having said this, as long as there is no contraindication to working, you can choose to continue. Some employers will request a letter from your obstetrician stating that you may continue working past 36 weeks.

WILL I BE PAID DURING MATERNITY LEAVE?

Employers are not required by law to pay employees during maternity leave. Some companies offer maternity benefit packages as part of their conditions of employment or as part of a collective bargaining agreement. These employer-provided benefits may include fully or partially paid maternity leave for several months, or may extend the period granted for maternity leave, as either unpaid or partially paid leave.

While on maternity leave you are eligible for UIF maternity benefits provided you have contributed to the fund for more than four months. These benefits range from 38 to 60 per cent of your average earnings over the last six months and are paid for a maximum of 121 days, or six weeks in the event of a miscarriage or a stillborn child. If you work less than 24 hours per week you are not eligible for benefits.

Providing the documentation required by the Department of Labour is tedious. There are private consultants who will assist you with your UIF application – they are usually well worth the fee they charge.

HINTS FOR THE OTHER HALF

- Be attentive and listen to your partner, so she feels safe and heard. She is possibly feeling large and unattractive, so remind her what you love and appreciate about her, and that you find her attractive.
- Your partner is very likely to be quite uncomfortable now, and massages, feet up, meals prepared and errands done for her will be hugely appreciated.
- Support her, tell her that she is doing an amazing job of nurturing your baby and be patient if she suffers from pregnancy brain and is rather forgetful at times.
- Ask her what she needs from you; don't guess or assume you are supposed to know.
- An excellent book to read is *The Birth Partner* by Penny Simkin.
- Turn your mind to how you can prepare for the labour room – music playlist and player, cold drinks packed in the fridge, making yourself familiar with the hospital bag, what's in it, and where to find the things she'll need.
- Be sure you know who to call, and their telephone numbers, when labour starts.

The esSense of 33–37 weeks

- By the end of pregnancy you may start to feel the weight of your pregnant body in your joints and muscles with backache, pelvic pain and discomfort while sleeping.

- Your weight gain has slowed dramatically as you are eating less at meals and may experience uncomfortable heartburn after eating.

- If you don't feel your baby move, lie on your side for two hours and count the movements; there should be more than 10 movements in that time.

- Your baby is fully developed and is fattening up ready for birth. Her lungs will mature over this period so that she won't require assistance with breathing at birth

- You will be seeing your caregiver two-weekly or even weekly at this stage.

CHAPTER 12

38 weeks to birth

Your baby is now full term and while you may be holding out for that due date, you should know that only 4 to 5 per cent of babies are born on their due date. In fact, 85 per cent are born within two weeks (before or after) of their due date.

CARING FOR YOURSELF

You are now considered full term and could give birth any day. Your diet should continue to be small meals, although after your baby engages you may manage slightly bigger portions again. Looking ahead to your breast-feeding diet, you will need an extra 500 calories a day to meet the extra energy for feeding your newborn. This could be a small full-cream plain yoghurt, eight almonds, an apple and a handful of biltong. Increase your liquid intake in preparation for birth and breast-feeding.

Supplements
Continue your antenatal iron supplement now and while breast-feeding. Omega supplements may slightly increase the risk of bleeding. Follow your caregiver's advice on whether to stop these until after birth.

Weight gain
Your weight gain will have slowed significantly and you may experience a small amount of weight loss leading up to birth. In the first few weeks post birth you will probably lose about 60 to 90 per cent of what you gained during your pregnancy. Don't fixate on weight loss; continue to eat healthy food, and exercise.

Antenatal appointments
As your baby is full-term and especially if you go over 40 weeks, you will see your caregiver weekly and even twice a week at this stage.

ULTRASOUND
An ultrasound may be done to
- check the condition and function of the placenta;
- check the amount of amniotic fluid; and
- assess your baby's growth.

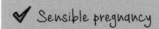

✔ Sensible pregnancy

Signs of labour

At this stage everything feels like a sign of labour and most first-time moms also worry that they won't recognise labour when it starts. You are probably in labour if:
- you have contractions that are increasingly uncomfortable and more regular. The interval between them becomes shorter and their duration increases (30-second contractions 5 minutes apart);
- a bloody show is passed. This mucous discharge mixed with blood is passed as the cervix starts to dilate and the mucous plug comes away;
- your waters break – you experience a gush of fluid that you have no control over. Sometimes it's just a small leak of fluid; wear a sanitary pad and consult your caregiver if it continues.

ALMOST READY FOR LABOUR

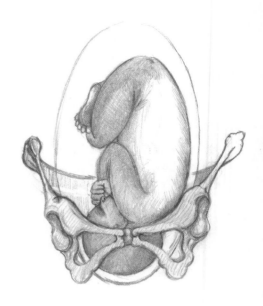

Your baby is head down

Almost all babies are head down by now. If your baby is still head up near the ribs (breech) or lying transverse, your caregiver may attempt to turn him (see p. 93). If he remains in this position, he will probably be delivered by C-section, which should be scheduled after 39 completed weeks.

Your baby engages

You may feel a sense of lightening as your baby's head moves downwards into the birth canal, creating a little more space below your ribs. This occurs when your baby engages (also called lightening or dropping).

Engagement refers to the process where your baby's head enters the pelvis – the head is engaged when at least half of it has moved into the pelvis.

This happens towards the end of pregnancy or in labour, but the timing is variable, and not every woman is aware of it.

As a rule of thumb, the baby's head should engage in the last two to three weeks of pregnancy in Caucasian women in their first pregnancy. In subsequent pregnancies, and in women of other race groups, specifically African women, engagement may only occur in labour.

Cervical changes

The cervix has been firmly closed and elongated and must change to allow your baby to pass through. These changes include softening and shortening (effacement). The uterus tilts and with it the cervix moves to become aligned with the vagina.

Again, timing of these changes, and the time taken for them to occur, varies.

If you and your caregiver have to make a decision on whether to induce labour, your caregiver will check whether all these cervical changes have occurred.

Signs you are close to labour

Shortly before you go into labour, you may experience some of these signs:

- **Energy spurt** You may have a couple of days of feeling very energetic, which may be ascribed to a nesting instinct – you want to make sure everything is ready for your baby.
- **Frequent loose stools or diarrhoea** This may be your body's way of preparing the space for your baby to move through the birth canal.
- **Lightening** Your baby drops down into your pelvis (engages) and there is less pressure under your ribs but more pressure on your pelvis.
- **Weight gain stops** and you may even lose some weight.
- **Increased Braxton Hicks contractions** As your uterus starts to prepare for labour, it practises by contracting intermittently. These contractions are generally not painful and you should be able to talk comfortably while they are happening.

Be patient

Don't worry about trying to bring on labour. Labour is initiated by your baby – wait for him. There is no scientific evidence that natural induction methods work. Medical induction should only be performed if necessary (see Chapter 14, p. 127).

Natural induction involves activating small amounts of labour hormones that will only be released when the time is right anyway. After 39 weeks, there is no harm in trying these:
- Drinking raspberry leaf tea
- Eating spicy foods
- Sensual kissing, nipple stimulation and having sex
- A brisk walk

If the due date has passed

Your due date is an estimate, usually calculated as 280 days from the first day of the last menstrual period. Clearly, you won't necessarily go into labour on this day. Only about 4 per cent of women go into labour on their due date. The normal range of pregnancy is 37 to 42 completed weeks. If this is your first pregnancy, your baby is more likely to be born after the due date. In second or subsequent pregnancies it is just as likely that your baby will come after the due date as before. The due date is often quite an emotional day; it's that date you've been working towards the entire pregnancy, but do remember these statistics if you're feeling a little despondent.

GOING OVERDUE

There are some risks if you go more than 7 to 10 days over your due date. You need to understand these risks so that you can be part of the decision-making process with your caregiver, who may suggest inducing (bringing on) labour.

Placenta The placenta ages with time and becomes less efficient at delivering nutrients and oxygen to the baby. It is reassuring if your placenta is functioning well and your baby continues to grow.

Passing meconium As your baby matures so do his intestines, and this means there is an increased likelihood that he will pass meconium, or baby poo – which is sterile (clean), and discolours the amniotic fluid yellow or green. If he does pass meconium, there is a risk that he will inhale the meconium-stained fluid at birth, which can cause a serious chemical pneumonia. Steps will be taken to prevent this

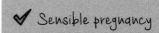

✔ **Sensible pregnancy**

When to call your caregiver
Reasons to call your caregiver remain the same as in the previous stage of pregnancy.

Warning signs of preeclampsia:
- Severe headaches
- Changes in vision – either blurred vision or flashing lights
- Severe pain in the upper abdomen, below the ribs
- Vomiting
- Sudden onset of swelling of the face, hands or feet

If these occur, you need to have your blood pressure and urine checked the same day.

Bleeding
You need to seek medical attention immediately if bleeding occurs that is:
- not associated with the mucous plug coming away;
- more than light spotting;
- accompanied by pain.

Your baby moving a lot less
If you don't feel foetal movements or there is a noticeable decrease in your baby's movements, these should be reported the same day.

by suctioning the fluid from your baby's nose and mouth at birth. This complication is more common in overdue babies. In rare cases a baby inhales meconium before delivery.

Baby grows Since your baby continues to grow, there is an increased chance of C-section as it may be more difficult to birth a larger baby naturally.

More serious risks While still very rare, there is an increase in the chance of stillbirth when you go over due date. The incidence of unexplained stillbirth is 1 in 3 000 at 37 weeks of pregnancy, but increases to 3 in 3 000 by 42 weeks. There is also an increased incidence of cerebral palsy in babies born after 42 weeks.

WHAT TO DO IF YOU ARE OVERDUE?
Whilst 42 completed weeks is traditionally taken to be the normal length of human pregnancy, many caregivers will advocate induction of labour when you are 7 to 10 days past due date to reduce these risks.

Should you choose not to induce labour, more frequent monitoring of your baby is recommended – at least twice a week past 42 weeks, with electronic foetal heart rate monitoring (cardiotocography or CTG), and ultrasound assessment of amniotic fluid volume. However, it is also important to understand that monitoring does not predict sudden events, like stillbirth.

Birth by C-section
If you are going to have your baby delivered by planned C-section for any reason, it is usually scheduled before onset of labour but, unless there is a medical reason, it should not be before 39 weeks.

It is often suggested that, if it is not an emergency and no precautions are required for your baby at birth, it is best to wait until labour starts before having your C-section. In this way, you allow your baby to show you when he is ready to be born.

In the following circumstances you will not be allowed to go into labour:
• Placenta lying over the cervix
• Breech or transverse presentation

The choice to await spontaneous labour is not without a downside. A large team is involved in a C-section and teamwork is what makes it the optimal experience for you and your baby. There could be some delay in performing the C-section, you might get a less motivated or prepared team than the one your obstetrician chooses to work with. Your obstetrician might not be available. In some cases, this can make a significant difference.

BECOMING A MOM

You are excited to meet your newborn. Remember that he may not look exactly as you have envisaged. He may be chubby or have wrinkly skin because he has started to lose the vernix that was protecting his skin from the wet water world of the womb. You may be besotted at first sight, or you may be tired and in pain and just want to sleep after birth.

Weekly progress

WEEK	Your baby's development	Your changing body
38	Your baby continues to grow and is about 49,8cm now. All his organs are ready to survive outside the womb. Tear ducts form in this last stage of pregnancy. Your baby's eye colour is genetically determined already but because babies eyes get darker after birth, it will be a few weeks or even months before you know his true eye colour. If he has brown eyes at birth they will probably stay brown but blue eyes can get darker and turn to green or brown by nine months old. He now knows your voice and the familiar taste and smell of your body.	Your cervix starts to soften in preparation for dilating or opening up.
39	Like adults, babies differ in length within a range of 46 to 56 cm but the average full-term baby is 51 cm. Your baby's fingernails keep growing and may extend over his fingertips at birth, especially if he goes over due date. The vernix – that white waxy coating that covered him for most of the pregnancy – will begin to be absorbed from now on. If he is born this week, you will notice that this vernix is still evident especially in his body creases – at his hips, neck and under his arms. Your baby is ready to be born and initiates labour when the time is right. Your baby's immunity is developing and, along with magical colostrum (early breast milk) in the days after birth, will set him up to be healthy for at least the first six months.	You are tired of waiting and are filled with excitement about meeting this precious new life. Your baby will likely have engaged by this week and this makes your pelvis more uncomfortable, increasing the need to urinate often.
40	Your full-term baby will weigh between 2,5 and 4,2 kg, with the average being 3,4 kg for boys and 3,2 kg for girls. Your baby has fattened up so he will look like a soft, rosy bundle at birth. He has all the movements of a newborn and like a newborn derives great pleasure from sucking his thumb. There are more touch receptors in and around the mouth, making this an important area for self-soothing.	A small percentage of babies arrive on their due date but if this is your first pregnancy you are likely to go past 40 weeks. As your cervix softens, a mucous plug may be released, indicating that your baby's birth is close.
41	As your baby is one week over due date and most of his vernix has been absorbed, his skin may be a little dry if he is born this week or next.	You visit your caregiver twice a week to monitor your precious baby's status and that of the placenta too. If labour doesn't start naturally this week, your caregiver will probably suggest that labour is induced.

WEEK	Your baby's development	Your changing body
42		Owing to increased risks if pregnancy is prolonged beyond 42 weeks, you will be preparing for delivery if your baby has not arrived.

Things to do

- **Monitor your baby's movement**. Keep monitoring your baby's movements and call your doctor if you are concerned that his movements have changed over a 24-hour period.
- **Set up a WhatsApp group** for news on your labour and the birth of your precious baby.
- **Savour the last moments** of being a couple and a woman without the commitments of a new baby. It's precious time – embrace the calm.

Frequently asked questions

Modern monitoring techniques give us useful information about the changes that occur during pregnancy and in labour. To be part of your decision-making process in birth, it is important to know what is normal and therefore does **not** require any intervention.

IS THERE ENOUGH AMNIOTIC FLUID?

There is a normal reduction in the amount of amniotic fluid with time and this is of no concern if your baby's growth is normal and the fluid measurement is more than 5 cm.

WHAT IS PLACENTAL CALCIFICATION?

As the placenta ages, there will be some calcification of the tissue, which shows up bright white on ultrasound. This is normal after 37 weeks of pregnancy and, on its own, is not a reason for induction of labour.

IS MY BABY TOO BIG OR SMALL?

Babies are not all the same size and, as the due date approaches, the variation increases. In addition, ultrasound also has its limitations regarding accuracy. A 'big baby' is not necessarily a reason to have a C-section so exercise caution when considering induction or C-section on the basis of your baby's size.

There are clear guidelines as to what is bigger (or smaller) than average, and what is abnormally big (or small). As long as your baby's measurements lie in the normal range, there is nothing to worry about.

More important than your baby's size is his growth over time. If he is small but continues to grow adequately he is fine.

If your baby measures abnormally large, a cause such as maternal diabetes must be investigated and, if abnormally small, a placental problem must be excluded.

AM I TOO SMALL TO DELIVER MY BABY VAGINALLY?

There is no way to predict with any accuracy if your body is well suited to vaginal birth. While the size and shape of your pelvis are important factors, it can only be assessed during the process of labour. Your baby's 'fit' can also not be predicted as it depends not only on his size (this estimation is not always accurate anyway), but also on his position related to your pelvis, and how well his chin is tucked in.

Studies have shown that, even with sophisticated measurements of the mother's pelvis and expert assessment of the baby's size, predictions for labour were wrong as often as they were right.

An experienced obstetrician or midwife might suspect that there is an increased likelihood of your requiring a C-section. If you have prioritised a vaginal delivery your caregiver should not present size as a reason to have a C-section but allow you to prepare for a change in birth method should it be necessary.

While size alone is an inaccurate predictor, other factors might influence your decision one way or another. In certain cases, for example maternal diabetes, C-section is indicated for a baby above a certain weight to avoid the complication of the baby's shoulder blocking his passage through the birth canal.

SHOULD I BE WORRIED IF THE CORD IS AROUND MY BABY'S NECK?

If an ultrasound reveals that the cord is around your baby's neck you need not be concerned. Although the umbilical cord is your baby's lifeline (delivering oxygen and nutrients), it is specifically designed to stretch, allow movement and bend (the cord is coiled). The tough substance of the cord protects the blood vessels so it can also withstand a degree of compression.

Your baby and the umbilical cord are surrounded by fluid, allowing the cord to slip over body parts. At birth, the cord is frequently around the baby's neck and it will simply be slipped over the head, or cut if there is not enough space to do so, before the body is delivered.

The cord around the neck or any other body part is only a problem if it is compressed enough to reduce blood flow. If this is significant it will be detected as changes of the heart rate.

It is only considered problematic if the cord is wrapped around the neck more than once. If there is also reduced amniotic fluid, or your baby's growth has not been optimal, your caregiver will be more cautious. If this is the case your baby's heart rate will be carefully monitored throughout labour and C-section may be recommended.

HINTS FOR THE OTHER HALF

- You are now playing a waiting game, full of excitement, fear and impatience. Take your partner out for a last 'just the two of us' dinner.
- Make sure you're available and contactable at all times.
- Your partner will not be sleeping well, so help her to be more comfortable, massaging her feet and shoulders, and book her a last pre-baby massage, if this isn't your forte. You'll win lots of points if you book her in for a manicure and pedicure, too!
- Love, care, attentiveness and patience will win the day!

The esSense of 38 weeks to birth

- Your baby will most likely be in a head-down position and will soon descend into the birth canal, leaving you feeling a little more comfortable.

- At around this time, your cervix starts to prepare to dilate by softening and shortening. An increase in mucous discharge is common.

- Your baby is probably about 50 cm long and weighs in the vicinity of 3 kg. Do not worry if you are told he is a 'big baby' – measurements of baby's size are not only unreliable, they are also not an indication of the ease with which he can be delivered vaginally.

- If you are having a scheduled C-section, it should be performed after 39 completed weeks of pregnancy to ensure your baby is as mature as possible.

- Call your doctor if you experience sudden severe headaches, changes in your vision, severe pain in the upper abdomen, vomiting, sudden swelling or bleeding, or perceive less movement of your baby.

CHAPTER 13

In preparation

Aqeelah wakes from a dream, panicky and uncomfortably breathless. The panic is all to do with the dream about her birth. There are so many unknowns and Aqeelah has the sense that she isn't prepared enough. She has been reading a lot and is now looking forward to starting her antenatal classes, hoping that this will fill in all the gaps.

As she lies awake for the next hour, she wonders if she is fit enough and how she would manage the pain. Her mind turns to the nursery, which is still incomplete, and the bags of unwashed clothes she has bought or been given. She vows to start washing those clothes and checking her to-do list today. This panicky rush of thoughts kick-starts Aqeelah's nesting phase, which will intensify as labour approaches.

It is wise to prepare for birth and your baby in the same way as you would prepare for a marathon or other ambitious, physically and mentally challenging events. Your body needs training and preparation, and you need to feel mentally and emotionally up to the task.

PREPARING YOUR BODY

Like a fine-tuned machine, your body needs to be prepared for the road ahead.

Fitness preparation

Labour is an apt word to describe the birthing process, as it is hard work, but with the right training your body will be conditioned and prepared for the task. You need stamina and strength, and also a body that is conditioned to relax. Practising breathing control and rhythm is very useful. Exercise can also be used to encourage your baby into an optimal position for easier labour.

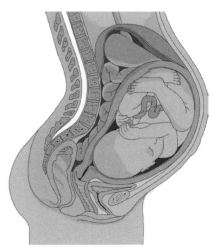

It is easier to birth a baby who is facing backwards (spine anterior) than one who faces forwards (posterior position). The following exercises may increase the likelihood of your baby's lying in an optimal position.

- Walking for 30 minutes each day is excellent for fitness and if this is all you can manage, you will be well enough prepared.
- Yoga and Pilates improve stamina, strength and breathing control, and are excellent preparation for childbirth. Yoga squats and poses such as the low lunge pose, cat stretch, child's pose and goddess pose are fabulous for opening the pelvis and moving your baby into the optimal anterior position.
- Swimming is excellent and, in addition to being non weight-bearing, has the benefit of being aerobic, using a large number of muscle groups and teaching good breathing control and rhythm.
- If you run or go to gym you can continue as long as you stay within your comfort zone, listen to your body and don't overheat or become dehydrated.
- After 30 weeks ease off on core strengthening, as your lower abdomen needs to relax and stretch to prepare for the birth, rather than tighten up.
- Exercises to help your baby to move into an anterior position include tilting your hips forward – a good way to do this is by leaning forward; you can do this leaning against a kitchen counter or sitting on a chair facing backwards or physio ball with your pelvis tilted. Going onto all fours and alternately arching and flattening your back is also a very good exercise to help your baby to move into this position.

Preparing for breast-feeding

No preparation of your breasts is required. Your nipples don't need toughening up and you are more likely to damage them if you try. If you have had breast surgery and would like to breastfeed it is helpful to see a lactation consultant before delivery, so that she can assess your chances of breast-feeding, and be on standby as you are more likely to need help in the first week. It is advisable to see her by day 4 after birth so that she can advise you if your milk isn't coming in adequately.

Preparing your perineum

The perineum is the area between the anus and the vagina. The physiological changes of pregnancy enable it to stretch to allow your baby's head through.

Perineal massage has been suggested to further increase the elasticity of the perineum and limit the risk of tearing or needing an episiotomy. An Epi-no is a device designed with a similar effect. Research has not shown that either of these methods is effective – do them if it helps you feel better prepared, but don't worry if you're not comfortable with it!

Perineal massage is done for five minutes a day, three to four times a week, from 36 weeks. After a warm, relaxing bath, lie semi-reclined, with pillows for comfort on your bed. Ensure you have clean hands and a mirror to see what you are doing. Put lube or oil on your thumbs, fingers and perineum. Place your thumbs up to the first knuckles inside the vagina, pressing down towards the rectum, with your fingers on your buttocks. Gently but firmly massage with your thumbs in a circular, repetitive movement for four to five minutes, also massaging from inside to out, as the baby would come out. There should be a stretching discomfort, but no pain or bruising. Breathe, practising your labour breathing technique, and consciously relax.

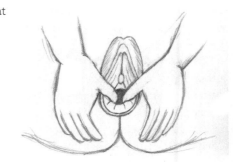

Preparing your pelvic floor

The muscles, ligaments and fascia of your pelvic floor support your internal organs, particularly your bowel, bladder and uterus. Pressure of the baby during pregnancy and relaxation from the pregnancy hormones can result in the pelvic floor's losing elasticity. Strengthening your pelvic floor can:

- prevent stress incontinence (urine leaking) during and after pregnancy;
- prevent prolapse of the bladder or uterus later in life;
- prevent vulval or anal varicose veins (haemorrhoids or piles);
- enable better control during delivery, so that you can relax these muscles when bearing down in the second stage.

How to do this

- Pilates and yoga strengthen and stabilise your core and pelvic floor muscles.
- Squatting and performing **Kegel exercises** (to your labour breathing rhythm) are helpful. Kegel exercises entail alternately tightening and relaxing the pelvic and vaginal muscles as you would if you were stopping urine mid stream. Practise them while stationary at a traffic light or while standing in a queue – tightening for five seconds then relaxing for five seconds, four or five times in a row.
- Avoid constipation by eating plenty of fibre.

As you approach labour, turn the emphasis from tightening this area, to allowing the relaxation and stretching to enable the birthing process to occur naturally.

PREPARING FOR BIRTH

Antenatal classes

Antenatal or birth preparation classes are an important part of preparing for birth and are a good way to help your partner feel involved. You will get not only practical information about labour and birth but, also support, a network of friends and shared excitement about the journey ahead. The friendships developing from your class will be part of your parenting journey for years to come.

A good antenatal class should cover:
- What to expect in the different stages of labour
- What is happening to your body during labour
- How to recognise labour and when to head to hospital or call your caregiver
- Delivery options and what the indications are for each
- Guidance on choices for you and your baby
- What to expect in terms of pain in labour and how you can use pain-relief options
- Medical procedures you may need in the birth process
- Establishing breast-feeding and the early days of feeding
- General parenting advice for the early days
- Partner support and preparing for parenthood.

CHOOSING A CLASS

Choose a class and teacher that resonate with your values. Be conscious of the type of delivery you want and choose a group that supports your intent and empowers that decision, e.g. if you are leaning towards an active natural birth versus an elective C-section you may choose different classes. It's also essential that there is a non-judgemental approach that embraces individual preferences and needs.

Attend a class in your area, so that you can easily meet up with the other new moms once your babies are born and offer practical support to one another. WhatsApp groups are fabulous for keeping housebound moms connected and feeling less alone, so it's worth getting one started within your antenatal class. These groups are also a lifesaver when you feel lonely, feeding in the middle of the night, and discover another mom or two awake and feeding or settling their baby, too.

There are many types of classes:
- **Independent midwife or childbirth educator** classes cover the basics of birth and pain management, and also touch on the early weeks with your baby.
- **Hypnobirthing classes** focus on natural pain relief methods including visualisation, hypnosis and relaxation methods and will empower you with strategies that are not covered in enough detail in most antenatal classes. They usually don't cover breast-feeding and care of your newborn baby.
- **Hospital-based classes** often emphasise hospital policy rather than individual choice, so may not be as independent as you may want but will give you a sense of what to expect at that hospital.
- **Online classes** For those who cannot attend a group class, there's an excellent South African online course: www.just-engage.com.
- **Weekends away** work well if you can't schedule weekly courses or have left it until the last minute.
- **One-on-one classes**, or online classes, might be preferred if you are more of a private person or have an unusual situation and don't want the group experience.

Hospital tour

If you are birthing in a hospital it's well worth doing the maternity ward tour. Find out when your hospital offers them. You can get a feel for the atmosphere and how things are done at your hospital. It will relieve your anxiety, knowing what to expect when you come in during labour.
- You will see the admission room, birthing rooms, waiting room, nursery and neonatal unit, kitchen and postnatal rooms.
- Enquire about hospital policies. Some don't allow dads to stay through the night after delivery or allow only one companion with a labouring mom.
- Ask to see their equipment – check if they have Pilates balls, birthing stools, and baths.
- You will also meet some of the staff and get a sense of how they work.
- Try to ascertain what paperwork can be done ahead of time and what you will be expected to do on the day.
- Ask if they have a lactation specialist.

Hospital bag

With one month to go it will be time to pack your bag for hospital. These are the items you will need:
- Medical scheme card, if applicable
- Toiletries such as toothbrush, toothpaste, hairbrush, creams, deodorant
- Maternity pads and panties
- Feeding bra
- Make-up
- Socks
- Snacks – nuts or dried fruit

- Nightie or pyjamas or yoga pants, a button-down shirt or breast-feeding top
- Speaker or earphones for your playlist
- Mirror
- Lip balm
- Outfit for going home
- Baby clothes (vest, socks, beanie and baby-grow) and swaddling blanket
- Eye shield
- Small portable nightlight
- Aromatherapy oils and electric burner

PREPARING YOUR LIFE

It is one thing to be prepared to give birth but the truth is that the birth will all be over in a matter of hours and, as significant as it is for you and your baby, the real outcome of a pregnancy is not the birth of the baby but the baby herself.

Adjusting to motherhood is significant and it is worth spending a little time turning your mind to the things that will make this easier.

Your home

Your baby will fit pretty seamlessly into your home until she is mobile, when you will suddenly find that you will be modifying your home quite dramatically. With a view to the first six weeks, this is what you need to consider:

SLEEP SPACE

Your baby needs a safe, consistent and calming place to sleep. This may be in your room or her own room. Listen to your gut preference regarding her sleep space rather than the noise of other people's opinions. As long as you can hear your baby and meet her needs timeously, it does not matter which room she sleeps in.

Have a crib as a consistent sleep space for at least one day-sleep and one night-sleep from birth. Since newborns sleep so often in the day, there will be times when she will sleep in the pram or car seat after a journey. Try to take her out of her car seat

---

SAFE SLEEP SPACE

Sleep marks the very first separation from your baby and you will be surprised at how much anxiety it causes. The risk of your baby not waking from a sleep (cot death or Sudden Infant Death Syndrome) is low, but because it is devastating and can happen, you do need to consider how to limit the risk as much as possible.

Millions are spent annually on SIDS research and, while the jury is still out on exactly what causes a baby to die in its sleep, we do know what the associated risk factors are. Co-sleeping on a soft surface, such as a couch, or a parent under the influence of drugs or alcohol, significantly increases the risk of death. A baby sleeping on her tummy likewise increases the risk. Smoking while pregnant and exposure to cigarette smoke is also seen as a risk factor.

Consider these important sleep safety tips:
- Soft materials, bedding, pillows or quilts should not be placed in the crib while your baby is sleeping. Your baby should not have any objects near or covering her face.
- Place your baby on her back or side to sleep. If you put your baby on her side, use a wedge to ensure she cannot roll onto her tummy.
- You may prefer a co-sleeper crib to allow for more convenient breast-feeding and contact while limiting the risk of SIDS.
- Avoid overheating your baby. It is not necessary to monitor the temperature in the room as long as it is comfortable for a lightly clothed adult.

when you arrive at a destination, as remaining in the curled-up position in a car seat for prolonged periods is not good for her physical development.

Feeding

In the early months you are going to spend many hours feeding. Make sure you have a comfortable chair in which to feed your baby. Place a little table next to the chair for your phone, a glass of water and your Kindle or a good book. If you have a toddler, a couch may work better so your older child can cuddle next to you and have a book read to him during feed times.

Pets

Make sure your pets (especially cats who love cuddling with a warm little body) cannot get into your baby's sleep space.

Shopping and cooking

While cooking meals in the first few weeks is going to be low on your priority list, nutritious meals are important to sustain your breast milk supply. Before your baby is born you should:

- stock up on basics like detergents, non-perishables and toilet paper;
- pre-make or buy frozen meals that can be taken out of the freezer on days when you just can't get a meal together;
- buy enough newborn and stage 1 nappies for two months – you have no idea how many you will go through (see p. 116).

Projects

If you are a busy executive, working woman or already a mother, there will be projects and tasks that need to be tied up before birth. Try as far as possible to leave one month before your due date with nothing to do. Finish work deadlines, buy presents for friends' kids and finish older children's projects ahead of time.

Urgent matters will come up in the last month, but having a clear plate will mean these are less stressful to deal with.

Products

You will be inundated with suggestions of items you simply 'have to have'. The truth is that when it comes to babies, less is more.

What you buy has everything to do with your budget and your desires, very little with need. If the chips are down, a few vests, baby-grows, blankets and lots of nappies are all your baby really needs. But, if you can afford some luxuries, here they are:

Clothes

Buy clothing that is 100 per cent cotton knit (stretchy) as this will help make dressing easier, is comfortable and aids your baby's temperature regulation.

Wash all new baby clothes and bedding before your baby arrives as factories often treat textiles with chemicals to make them feel or smell a certain way. Wash everything in a gentle detergent and instead of using a softener, which will have a fragrance, use white spirit vinegar (2 tablespoons in the softener section of the washing machine). Vinegar is a great softener and has no chemicals added and no fragrance once the clothes are dry.

In the early days, you need:
- Sleeveless vests for summer babies, long-sleeved for winter, and some baby-grows.
- If your baby spits up a lot, you will need more clothing and, once she starts teething, she will drool and need bibs to absorb the moisture.
- Summer babies need hats for hot days.
- In winter, you need beanies, fleecy jackets or onesies for the cold days.

TOILETRIES

Your baby's skin is a vital and fragile barrier. Certain products used unwisely on your baby in the early days can disrupt this natural barrier and in the long term contribute to allergies and irritation. Your baby's skin can also absorb chemicals, so the fewer chemicals in a cream, the better. Some chemicals affect your baby's own hormone system.

The choice is broad, but the principle is keep it simple. Don't swap lotions unnecessarily, use fragrance-free for the first three months and check the labels. Avoid products with dyes, parabens, sulphates and ethanol.

You need the following products:
- **Washing** Use simple fragrance-free aqueous cream rather than soap.
- **Moisturiser** Use fragrance-free moisturising cream such as Cetomacrogol (Epimax) for dry patches and eczema.
- **Nappy cream** Nappy cream is not needed with disposable nappies. If you are going to use a preparation to prevent chafing, use Milko balm. Cornstarch powder can be used if your baby has a red bum (not a full-blown nappy rash) to absorb the dampness and prevent nappy rash from developing. If your baby develops a nappy rash use a zinc-based nappy cream such as Sudocrem.
- **Nappies** With the environment in mind you may like the thought of not filling up our landfill sites with tons of nappies, but the carbon footprint when washing and drying reusable nappies is also considerable. Whatever you decide, it's worth using disposables for the first few weeks. The number of soiled nappies produced daily by a well-fed breast-fed baby for the first four weeks will intimidate the most courageous parents! You may be relieved to hear that the frequency of poos reduces for most by four to six weeks. If you use environmentally friendly nappies, you will do well to use disposables at night, as the reusables generally don't last through the night.
- **Cotton wool** pads or balls are good for cleaning your baby's face and bum.
- **Nappy wipes** These will come in handy for dirty hands and bottoms. Don't use wipes in the early weeks or when your baby has a nappy rash.

LINEN

Bed linen must be soft, preferably 100 per cent cotton or bamboo for temperature regulation.
- **Swaddle** You need some blankets or swaddles in a stretch cotton or muslin fabric.
- **Blankets** You may want to get a couple of warmer blankets to cover your baby when swaddled in colder weather and for trips out in the pram.
- **Sheets** Fitted sheets in soft cotton knit are best.
- **Sleeping bags** Your baby can be swaddled until she is rolling; thereafter move her into a sleeping bag for night sleeps so that she doesn't get cold if she kicks her blankets off.

FEEDING EQUIPMENT

Breast pumps range from basic hand pumps to hospital-grade double electric pumps, costing between a few hundred to a few thousand rand.

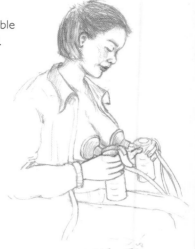

- A hand pump will do only for occasional pumping; it's not appropriate for exclusive pumping, as you may get a repetitive wrist injury.
- If possible, buy an affordable single or double electric pump. Bear in mind that you don't always get a better pump if you spend more money. Reviews and opinions of friends or clinic sisters are helpful for decision-making. If you are pumping at work or pumping more than once or twice a day, do get a double pump, as it empties both breasts at once, halving the expressing time.
- It's not advisable to share pumps or buy second-hand, unless they are closed system pumps and you each have your own handset. This is due to the danger of milk refluxing into the motor and being unhygienic. A pump also has a limited lifespan, so lending someone a pump for any length of time will shorten its lifespan.

Bottles Breast-fed babies may never use a bottle and might move directly onto a sippy cup closer to a year, but you may want to get one just in case you need it.
- If your baby is bottle-fed you will need six to eight bottles. By six weeks many babies are drinking more than 120 mℓ per feed, so it's worth mainly having 250 mℓ bottles.
- You need a smaller teat for water/breast milk (SS or S), and a slightly larger teat for formula (S, M or L), especially if you are using a thickened formula.

Steriliser You should sterilise all feeding equipment and dummies until your baby is moving and reaching (after six months). Microwave sterilisers are convenient and take roughly three minutes. Alternately boiling water or liquid sterilising solution can be used. Sterilising liquid can be used for several days before being changed. A small container of liquid steriliser is handy to leave your baby's dummies in when not being used, but do rinse before using items that have been in the sterilising solution.

NURSERY

The nursery is your baby's sleep space and needs to be soothing. Use the principles of the womb world:
- **Light** A light dimmer or night light is essential for night feeds so that she is not fully woken by bright light at night. Curtains or blinds with block-out lining will keep her sleeping better during the day and the early hours of the morning.
- **Colour** Keep the colours of her room muted and neutral – bright and contrasting colours are not what she is used to in the womb and may overstimulate her.
- **Sound** Music with a rhythm around 72 beats per minute is lulling, reminding her of your heartbeat. Likewise, a white noise machine or app is perfect for recreating the soothing womb space for sleep.
- **Temperature** While it's not necessary to rigidly monitor temperature, be mindful of the nursery's room temperature, so that it is comfortable for you, but not too warm for your baby. A sweaty baby who is pinker than usual needs less clothing and blankets. A humidifier will moisten the air and a wall panel heater will take off the chill in a cold room. A fan or air-conditioner will cool the room in summer. Gas heaters are not safe.

- **Smells** Neutral smells and fragrance-free items are best for the early days. You can sleep with her bed sheets for a couple of nights before she is born so that her sleep space smells of you when she sleeps in the crib in the early days.
- **Furniture** The most important items of furniture are a cot, a changing table with a changing mat, a comfortable chair for feeding and a shelf or side-table. Your newborn will sleep in a crib or a carrycot in her big cot. Make sure your furniture is coated with lead-free paint and that the changing station is at hip to waist height – this is really important for protecting your back.

TRAVEL

Travel system You will need a pram and car seat, often together in a travel system, ideally with Isofix.

> ### Making sense
> ....
> **Isofix** is an internationally standardised baby car seat fitting system, installed into all new cars worldwide since 2006. It increases the ease and safety of clipping in car seats securely.

Carrier Wearing your baby in a carrier is the best way to soothe her and still have your hands free – against your body, she gets all the benefits of your sensory world:
- Your smell
- Lulling movement
- Motor stimulation of her neck and back muscles
- Visual awareness of your world
- Eye contact
- The sounds of your heartbeat and voice up close

The choices:
- A ring sling or wrap carrier can be used from birth, for most of the first year. Make sure you can see your baby's face when she is in the sling and that her airway is not obstructed by the fabric.
- An upright pouch carrier can be used from two months onwards. For comfort it should carry most of the weight on your hips, rather than your shoulders. Shoulder straps should be wide and comfy, your baby's neck should be well supported and your baby held snugly against your body.

BABY MONITORS

While baby monitors are not essential, some parents find them useful and reassuring. Baby monitors can monitor sound, visuals and breathing.

Because they are prone to false alarms, these devices can increase anxiety, rather than decrease it, so are not recommended for everyone.

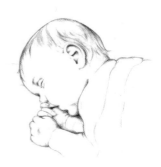

If your baby has been born prematurely or has had any episodes of apnoea, you may be advised to buy a breathing monitor. A movement sensor pad under the mattress or a portable monitor that clips onto your baby's nappy are both examples of breathing monitors.

Shopping list

Toiletries
- [ ] Aqueous cream
- [ ] Cetomacrogol or Sudocrem
- [ ] Milko balm
- [ ] Wecesin powder or surgical spirits for umbilical cord cleaning
- [ ] Ear buds
- [ ] Cornstarch powder
- [ ] Cotton-wool pads or balls
- [ ] A pack of wipes for later

Clothing
- [ ] 4–10 vests, short- and long-sleeved
- [ ] 4–7 baby grows
- [ ] 3–4 fleeces/jerseys
- [ ] 5 pairs of booties/socks
- [ ] 5 bibs
- [ ] 2 hats: beanies for the cold, sunhats to protect from sun

Linen
- [ ] 2–4 100% cotton stretch fabric sheets for each of your baby's sleep spaces – cot or carrycot
- [ ] 2 towels, hooded
- [ ] 2–6 muslin cloths
- [ ] 2–4 stretchy swaddling blankets
- [ ] 2–4 warmer blankets

Nappies
- [ ] 4 packs of newborn nappies or 15–20 reusable nappies
- [ ] Nappy sacks
- [ ] Nappy bag

Feeding
- [ ] Breast pump
- [ ] Breast pads
- [ ] 1–6 125/250 mℓ bottles
- [ ] Teats – silicone or latex

Accessories
- [ ] Dummies
- [ ] Microwave steriliser
- [ ] Steriliser liquid and container
- [ ] Bottlebrush
- [ ] Soft hairbrush

Nursery and outdoor equipment
- [ ] Cot or carrycot with new breathable mattress
- [ ] Changing station with waterproof changing mat
- [ ] Nappy bucket with bags
- [ ] Baby bath or bath seat
- [ ] Night-light
- [ ] Pram and car seat
- [ ] Baby sling or pouch

PREPARING YOUR MIND

Aside from preparing for birth and preparing for a baby, you need to prepare your mind to be a mom and there will be challenges along the way.

Practical decisions

During your pregnancy, you will have discovered that everyone has an opinion on your baby and your role as a parent. There are few areas in life where there are more 'experts' – all and sundry will be an expert on your baby.

Unfortunately other moms can be quite opinionated and unkind when their ideas do not coincide with one another's – try to shut out the noise and listen to your inner voice on these issues:

- Childbirth method (natural versus C-section)
- Circumcision
- Vaccination
- Co-sleeping
- Breast- versus bottle-feeding
- When and how to introduce solids
- Routine
- Crying
- Childcare
- Stay-at-home or working mom

It is very important that you make decisions, from childbirth to childcare, in a structured manner. This four-step approach works well:

1. Know your own mind – before researching or discussing anything, write down your own feelings on the matter.
2. Then discuss this with your partner.
3. Then consult one 'expert' voice – a website, a family member, a book or a clinic sister. Don't consult too many as you will get a lot of conflicting opinions.
4. Make your choice and be clear about your boundaries so as not to invite discussion.

Adjusting your mind and embracing these coping mechanisms can make the transition to parenthood easier:

1. **Let go**. Birth and mothering are about letting go. There is never a time in your life that flexibility and surrender are as important. Babies are not predictable and rigidity can lead to postnatal distress (PND) if you feel like a failure when things don't go according to plan.
2. **Adjust your expectations**. You will be overwhelmed, you won't have all the answers and your days will be unpredictable. If you have realistic expectations, your real-life experience will be less traumatic.
3. **Sleep**. You will be more exhausted than you can imagine and it will irritate you when people say, "Sleep when your baby sleeps." You will have no time to even shower and will resent having to use your precious 'free time' when your baby is asleep to sleep. But truly – it is something you must do – just once a day for 30 minutes and going to bed early will help you cope.
4. **Breathe deeply**. There will be people who will get under your skin with their unsolicited advice and unhelpful opinions. It is not worth making an enemy of your sister-in-law or falling out with your best friend – just smile and move on.
5. **Believe in yourself**. Insecurity will be your constant companion. You will second-guess yourself all the time. Media, 'experts' and well-meaning friends will seem to know more than you. But you need to know that you are your baby's mother and if you can listen to your gut feeling, it will lead you to make the right decisions for her.

And, finally, know this – women have survived birth for centuries, babies have survived inexperienced mothers forever and women grow into amazing moms with each generation. History says that you will survive this and thrive. Embrace your moment.

The esSense of preparation

* Preparing your body for birth entails becoming fit, preparing your perineum for the big stretch (if it makes you feel better prepared), and strengthening your pelvic floor muscles to support your pelvic organs – the uterus, bladder and bowel.

* Antenatal classes provide good preparation for labour and basic baby care.

* You need to prepare your home, pets and the people around you for a baby. A nursery and all the necessities need not be an expensive operation. Prioritise what is really essential.

* Preparing your mind for motherhood entails an enormous mind shift from control to letting go, from perfection to acceptance and from sanity to sleepless delirium.

CHAPTER 14

A guide to birth

Jenny calmly breathes in and out, coaxing Sascha through each contraction. She has not left Sascha's side for 18 hours and the final moment is here, the moment in which she will touch a new life and deliver Sascha's precious bundle to her chest. She takes a deep breath and recognises the momentous event that she is honoured to be part of – the birth of Sascha's baby.

Jenny's life calling was to be a midwife. It is not only because she loves babies; it is because she knows that this moment is a defining moment for women. All mothers remember their baby's birth for better or for worse. And each birth, whether by vaginal delivery, a water birth or C-section is precious. Each woman deserves to be held with kindness and respect. This is Jenny's gift to the women she cares for in labour and delivery.

You have consciously embraced your pregnancy journey and now here you are pondering birth. It is time to understand exactly what birth options you have. This chapter discusses all the options you are likely to be presented with. You can consider all these routes and put them into your birth plan to be discussed with your doctor or midwife at your next visit.

BIRTH OPTIONS

It is worth seeing your birth options on a continuum, from low intervention (a natural birth allowing nature to take its course), through to high intervention (a medicalised birth with interventions that make the process predictable).

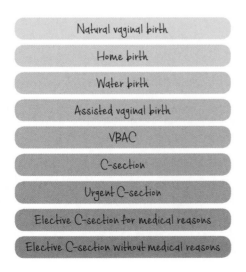

Natural vaginal birth

Home birth

Water birth

Assisted vaginal birth

VBAC

C-section

Urgent C-section

Elective C-section for medical reasons

Elective C-section without medical reasons

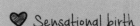 **Sensational birth**

However your baby is delivered, your birth should be very special. It is critical that you are part of the decision-making and feel that your voice is heard. You may choose, after reading this chapter, to go with low interventions and find along the way that you prefer to have an intervention, such as pain relief, or your birth method may change completely due to a medical situation. Understanding birth options and interventions will help you make sense of birth and facilitate your decisions and acceptance.

There are two distinct options for the delivery of your baby – a natural vaginal delivery or a C-section delivery. Within each category there are options:

Vaginal birth
- Natural vaginal birth
  » Vaginal home birth
  » Water birth
- Vaginal birth with interventions
- Vaginal birth after C-section (VBAC)

C-section
- Unscheduled or urgent C-section
- Elective C-section
- Gentle C-section

Vaginal birth

NATURAL VAGINAL BIRTH

Your body is designed to deliver your baby vaginally and natural vaginal delivery is more likely if you give birth without interventions. These include induction, artificial rupture of membranes, and assisted delivery such as forceps and vacuum extraction. Having to wear a hospital gown, being confined to a labour room and restricting your eating and drinking are also seen as unnecessary interventions. Routine shaving of pubic hair and administering enemas belong in the history books.

Intravenous therapy, continuous foetal monitoring and episiotomy might be indicated for medical reasons but should not be routine interventions.

You are likely to have a natural vaginal birth if you:
- have belief in your body's ability to give birth naturally;
- have a midwife-led delivery or an obstetrician who advocates natural delivery;
- prepare with good diet, exercise and antenatal classes, and have formulated your choice in a birth plan;
- stay at home until in active labour;
- have a doula present with you and a supportive partner;
- give birth in a relaxed, undisturbed place which may be at home, in a midwife-led maternity unit or at hospital;
- choose to walk around and not be limited to one room, wear what you want and labour in any position or in a bath.

VAGINAL HOME BIRTH

The environment in which you have your baby has been found to be an important factor in a normal physiological birth process. In a low-risk pregnancy, with a qualified and certified midwife and an accessible backup obstetrician, homebirth is an option and risks are few.

Your midwife, often accompanied by a doula, will not leave you and you will be able to labour in a familiar and relaxed space. Your midwife will have emergency equipment such as a drip and fluids for you and your baby, oxygen, emergency medication and airways suctioning, and ventilation equipment for your baby. There must always be a backup obstetrician on call should you need to transfer to hospital. For this reason most home births are planned to take place within 20 minutes of a hospital facility. If you need medical assistance, the hospital where your backup obstetrician works will be prepared ahead of your arrival.

You are likely to have a home birth if:

- you are secure in the knowledge that this natural process is within your capacity as a woman;
- you have a midwife as your caregiver;
- you have a low-risk pregnancy;
- you value privacy and a nurturing, familiar space to give birth in;
- you have prioritised a natural vaginal birth (without interventions).

Role of the doula

A doula is a birth companion who guides and supports you and your partner throughout labour and birth. Her support is emotional and physical, creating a safe and calm environment to allow labour to progress relatively uninterrupted. She reassures, comforts and encourages, and gives suggestions to ease distress and discomfort. Studies show that women attended by doulas during labour and birth have fewer interventions and better outcomes.

Your doula will not make decisions about the management of labour. She is there to support the decisions made by you and your midwife or obstetrician. Her support continues regardless, whether you choose to have an epidural, or delivery is by C-section.

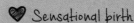

♥ Sensational birth

Why choose vaginal delivery?

- Uncomplicated vaginal birth has the lowest risk to the mother.
- The baby is less likely to have respiratory distress at birth.
- There is less chance of separation of Mom and Baby after birth.
- It is a better start to breast-feeding.
- There are potentially a lower risk of digestive issues such as allergies and obesity later.
- You have a more alert baby after birth owing to labour hormones.
- You avoid surgery and its complications.

WATER BIRTH

Water birth is a very specific and personal choice where part or all of the labour and birth process occurs in a bath of warm water. This can be in a hospital, birthing centre or home setting. Being immersed in warm water is an excellent pain-relief technique and labouring in water is a positive experience, whether you give birth there or not.

Giving birth in water can be a safe option and may have benefits such as shorter labour, fewer episiotomies, less pain medication and fewer epidurals, more likelihood of an intact perineum with no increased risk for your baby. You may also have a calmer labour. As long as the water temperature and your baby's heart rate are carefully monitored he won't take his first breath immediately and he will continue to receive oxygen via the umbilical cord for a short while until he is lifted out of the water. (For detailed, evidence-based information, go to http://evidencebasedbirth.com/waterbirth/.)

PAIN RELIEF AND WATER BIRTH

Water provides buoyancy and relaxes the body and can be used in the first stage of labour as a natural pain relief. Because it relaxes you and reduces pain it can speed up the first stage of labour. If you give birth in water you are less likely to need pain relief. If you do need more relief than the water is providing, you can use gas, but not a transcutaneous electrical nerve stimulation (TENS) machine or epidural.

Approach the possibility of a water birth with an open mind, rather than something to be insisted upon, as you may be disappointed. Your labour needs to be completely smooth sailing for you to stay in the water for the birth process. Also be prepared to leave the water after your baby is born, as the placenta is best delivered out of the water, so that post-partum bleeding can be monitored.

It is vital that your midwife or obstetrician is trained in water-birth technique and that you use the right equipment. There is an increased risk of infection for your baby if the bath isn't properly cleaned. There is also a risk of water inhalation if the delivery of the baby is delayed, or foetal distress has not been picked up.

Careful preparation is essential for a water birth. You need:
- A large, deep, birthing bath (can be rented) in a warmed room
- Clean water at 36 to 37 degrees C
- Water thermometer
- Waterproof foetal heart-rate monitor
- Blankets and towels prepared for when Mom and Baby leave the water.

VAGINAL BIRTH WITH INTERVENTIONS

You prioritise natural birth but are open to the interventions that modern medical science offers. You may be open to induction at or around your due date, medical pain management during labour, and the option of an epidural.

Intervention is more likely if:
- you are set on not going over your due date;
- you are induced with medication or have your membranes artificially broken;
- you would prefer to limit your pain and have requested an epidural;
- you give birth in a private hospital;
- you want a specific obstetrician to deliver your baby meaning less flexibility on delivery date if your doctor is not on call or is away;
- you labour in one position, particularly on your back;
- you head to hospital very early on in labour.

VAGINAL BIRTH AFTER C-SECTION (VBAC)

You might be a candidate for VBAC if you had only one previous C-section. Having had a previous C-section does limit your options, but VBAC is considered a safe option if there are no contraindications and labour is managed appropriately. Not all obstetricians support VBAC, either because of perceived risks or because of concern that the facilities are not adequate for the increased monitoring and interventions that may be required. Success rates for VBAC vary considerably, with some obstetricians reporting a 72 to 75 per cent success rate and others not offering VBAC as an option at all. It is a more labour-intensive option for midwives and obstetricians.

There is a risk of rupture of the uterus (0,5 per cent of VBACs), which is a serious complication that can be fatal for Mother and Baby. Because of the risks you will be assessed for suitability for VBAC.

VBAC must take place in a suitably staffed hospital with facilities for an urgent C-section and neonatal resuscitation, and you will be advised to have an intravenous drip and continuous electronic foetal monitoring once you are in active labour.

You can consider a VBAC if:
- you are carrying one baby (not twins or more);
- your baby is positioned head down;
- you have only had one previous C-section;
- your previous C-section incision (cut) was transverse (from left to right) in the lower part of the uterus (a lower segment C-section).

Birth by Caesarean section

A C-section is a surgical operation to deliver your baby via a cut into the lower abdomen. It can be **elective** (planned – usually occurring before labour starts) or **unscheduled/urgent** (taking place once labour has started, usually where vaginal birth was planned).

URGENT C-SECTION

Emergency C-Section is unscheduled and becomes necessary when vaginal birth poses a risk for you or your baby.

You may need an urgent C-section if:

- you experience bleeding during pregnancy or birth caused by separation of the placenta from the uterine wall (*abruptio placentae*);
- you have significant bleeding from placenta praevia;
- your baby's head isn't making adequate progress through the pelvis because of size, position or both, despite adequate time and adequate contractions (cephalo-pelvic disproportion);
- your baby is in foetal distress, indicated by his heart rate, and there may be evidence of meconium (baby poo) in the amniotic fluid;
- you are in labour but your baby is lying breech or transverse;
- the cord slips out of the cervix below your baby's head and there is a risk of its being squashed, resulting in a lack of oxygen to your baby (cord prolapse);
- you have complications such as eclampsia – seizures resulting from preeclampsia (high blood pressure).

ELECTIVE C-SECTION FOR MEDICAL REASONS

A C-section will be planned when necessitated by conditions of the pregnancy.

You are likely to have an elective C-section for medical reasons if:

- you are having a planned premature delivery;
- continuing with your pregnancy is a risk to you (e.g. preeclampsia/high blood pressure), or your baby (e.g. baby not growing owing to a placental problem);
- you have a multiple pregnancy;
- your baby is in an abnormal position – C-section is always recommended for a transverse lie and usually for a breech presentation;
- your placenta lies over the cervix (*placenta praevia*) or other placenta complications;
- you have had two or more C-sections before;
- your baby is abnormally large, which increases the risk of the baby's shoulder blocking the birth canal. This is most often a concern in diabetic mothers with a baby who is estimated to weigh over 4 kg.

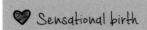

♥ Sensational birth

Is C-section safer?
While the reasons given for a C-section generally revolve around safety, the truth is that a C-section for medical reasons is needed in fewer than one in four births. Performing a C-section when it is not necessary carries a higher risk than natural birth.

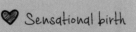

♥ Sensational birth

Balancing the value of C-section
A C-section is a birth safety net and a life-saving intervention when needed. If you are told that you need a C-section owing to a medical emergency, even when it is not what you planned and wanted, it is important that you make the mental adjustment and accept that this is the best course of action for you and/or your baby.

ELECTIVE C-SECTION WITHOUT MEDICAL REASONS

Like most things in life, there are pros and cons to both vaginal birth and C-section. You have the power to choose to have a C-section and feel good about your decision, even if it is not medically necessary. It is not a second-rate birth and if it is planned it will be beautiful and as special as a natural delivery.

Your decision is a personal one and will depend on your history, your expectations, the conditions of this pregnancy and your plans for future pregnancies. Unless there is a definite medical reason for a C-section, or alternatively why it should be avoided, your caregiver should provide you with facts that you can use to make your own choice.

If you are not sure how you want to give birth, it is often best to wait and see how the pregnancy pans out – the decision might become easier later on.

Having an elective C-section without medical reason has advantages and risks you need to consider.

	Risks of C-section	**Advantages of a planned C-section**
Risk to baby versus convenience	Delivery too early can result in an increased risk of breathing problems and difficulty latching. Elective C-sections should not be performed before 39 completed weeks unless there is a medical reason.	Knowing the date creates convenience and efficiency.
Risk of complications	All surgery has an inherent risk of infection, bleeding and damage to other organs for the mother. Although a low risk, it is greater than with vaginal delivery.	A lower chance of complications with a planned C-Section than an emergency C-section as potential complications of labour are avoided. Most C-sections are done under regional (spinal or epidural) anaes-thetic, which is a particularly safe form of anaesthesia.
Mom's emotional state	You may feel criticised for having a second-rate birth and need to manage these feelings to be secure in your choice.	If you have a phobia of birth, having a C-section can help manage these fears. Discuss it with your caregiver to be sure that you are making the correct choice.
Reproductive and pelvic organ health	A small increased risk of *placenta praevia* and *placenta accreta* in women who have several C-sections (usually more than four). These are serious complications with a risk of haemorrhage and hysterectomy. If planning a larger family you should avoid C-section where possible.	Avoids the risk of vaginal tears and episiotomy and may reduce the risk of pelvic organ prolapse.

HOW BIRTH AFFECTS PELVIC ORGAN PROLAPSE

Being pregnant and giving birth are risk factors for pelvic organ prolapse (e.g. the bladder 'dropping' and pushing against the vaginal wall). It is not clear if having a C-section reduces this risk. Many factors are involved in pelvic organ prolapse (for example, the inherent connective tissue strength) and these might be more important than type of delivery.

Vaginal birth is associated with an initial increased likelihood of stress incontinence. With time, the difference between vaginal birth and birth by C-section isn't evident.

Assisted delivery (specifically forceps delivery) and large babies also increase the risk of pelvic organ prolapse.

What a C-section involves

This is what you can expect when delivering by C-section:

You will require anaesthetic, almost always regional anaesthesia (spinal or epidural), as it is the safest form of anaesthetic for you and your baby and you will be awake to experience and participate in the birth.

An intravenous drip is necessary, as is a urinary catheter to empty your bladder. It will be inserted once your anaesthetic is in place. Your vital signs will be monitored during the procedure – usually by means of a blood pressure cuff on your arm, a monitor on one finger to measure the oxygen saturation of your blood, and electrodes on your chest to monitor your heart activity.

WHO IS PRESENT?

- Your partner (or someone chosen by you as support) should always be allowed.
- An anaesthetist will administer the anaesthetic and remain present throughout, and is assisted by an anaesthetic nurse.
- Your obstetrician will perform the surgery, assisted by a second doctor.
- A scrub sister assists the surgeon with instruments and equipment.
- Another floor nurse fetches and carries and counts swabs and instruments.
- A paediatrician will see to your baby and will have a nurse (usually a midwife) to assist.

THE PROCESS

Once your anaesthetic has taken effect, your abdomen will be cleaned with antiseptic and covered with sterile drapes, exposing only the surgical site. A screen is placed at the level of your chest – usually neither you nor your partner will see the surgery.

A 10-cm incision is made along your bikini line. The abdominal wall will be stretched to make space for the baby. The assistant will press on your abdomen to deliver the baby. You will be aware of movement and pressure and may be surprised by the amount of effort it requires to deliver your baby.

Your baby will be delivered very soon after the start of surgery. The surgeon will show you your baby before the paediatrician checks that all is well, in which case your baby will be given to you wrapped in a warm towel. Unless your baby needs special care, he can usually remain with you for the duration of the surgery. Some units routinely transfer the baby to the nursery – ask about this.

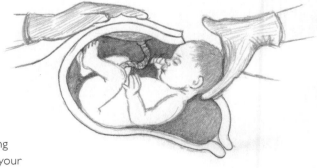

After surgery, you will be kept in a recovery area for 20 to 30 minutes to ensure that you are stable before you are transferred you back to the ward. Depending on routines at the hospital where you deliver, your baby may or may not remain with you here.

Your drip and catheter will remain in place, and you will require pain medication as the regional anaesthetic wears off.

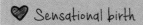

Sensational birth

Natural or gentle C-section

C-section is major abdominal surgery and your and your baby's safety remains the most important focus. But you can safely have a gentler C-section birth by replicating a natural delivery with all or some of these arrangements:

• The monitors to track your vital signs can be placed on your body on the sides of your chest so that they do not interfere with you holding your baby on your chest once he is born. Ask for the pulse monitor to be removed from your finger once your baby is born so you can stroke him. Some monitors can be attached to your legs rather than arms.

• Your surgeon and anaesthetist will require adequate light to work by but ask to dim the lights over your head once surgery starts so that your baby will be in gentle light once he is with you.

• Awareness by the staff that this is a special once-only time for you should reduce background noise and chit-chat.

• Play music of your choice – ascertain whether you need to bring a device to play the music.

• The screen, which is usually at the level of your chest and blocks your views of surgery, can be lowered at the time of delivery so you can see your baby being born if you prefer.

• You may request delayed cord clamping (see p. 141).

• Your hospital gown can be loosened so that you can hold your baby closer to your skin.

• Once your baby is born, he can be placed on your chest for immediate skin-to-skin contact.

• Have the paediatrician check his condition while he lies on your chest, assuming he is well and requires no assistance.

When discussing these possibilities with your obstetrician and paediatrician, safety is always the most important factor. Surgery is also not always predictable and some requests may not be possible if surgery or anaesthesia doesn't go according to plan.

IF YOUR BABY ARRIVES BEFORE YOU GET TO HOSPITAL

It's every mom and dad's worst nightmare – what happens if we don't get to the hospital in time? It's highly unlikely, but to take the drama out of it, know that not much skill is required if all is well. It helps to have a couple of towels, but that's about all you need.

If Mom is pushing and the baby's head is coming out on your way to the hospital or birthing centre, stop driving and help her. Ensure she is positioned so that the baby can come out freely and safely.

Hold a towel at the perineum to receive the baby so he doesn't drop out and encourage the mom as she's pushing, telling her what you can see and that all is well. Once the baby is born place her on the mom's naked abdomen, where he can stay warm.

If the membranes haven't ruptured, pull them off your baby's face, so he can breathe, dry him and look for encouraging signs of life – a pink, tensed body rather than a blue or limp baby. A crying baby tells you all is well! Don't clamp and cut the cord; just leave it be – it will stop pulsating in three to five minutes. Keep Mom and Baby warm as you get them to hospital for the placenta to be delivered.

If it's not possible to get to a hospital wait for signs that the placenta has separated (blood coming from the vagina) and gently pull the cord while Mom pushes the placenta out. Then it's important to rub the uterus and check that it is tight and hard, like a tennis ball, below her belly button (umbilicus). This will prevent excessive bleeding. More than a cup of blood loss means you do need to get to a hospital immediately for medical attention.

INTERVENTIONS DURING LABOUR AND BIRTH

You need to know about interventions that take place before, during and after birth. Some are more invasive than others and in some cases the decision may be out of your hands. Many have been developed for high-risk pregnancies and are life-saving (C-section) or pain-relieving (epidural) interventions. Others are simply interventions that make a medical team's life a little easier and have resulted in a medicalised approach to birth (putting on a hospital gown and keeping a patient on the bed). An uncomplicated birth can and should occur without any interventions.

From the start of labour to birth there are several potential interventions.

inducing labour → rupturing membranes → enema → hospital gown → keeping you on the bed → IV line → foetal monitoring → episiotomy → forceps/vacuum delivery → epidural → c-section

Inducing labour

As you approach 38 weeks, you become increasingly uncomfortable and impatient to meet your baby. It's not surprising many women become preoccupied with how to start labour.

As the end of pregnancy approaches, your cervix ripens; it changes from rigid and closed with a long neck, becoming softer and more pliant so that it shortens and dilates in response to increasing uterine contractions. Induction entails encouraging the cervix to ripen and, once the cervix is ripened, rupturing the membranes, which frequently initiates contractions.

If contractions are inadequate, oxytocin can strengthen them.

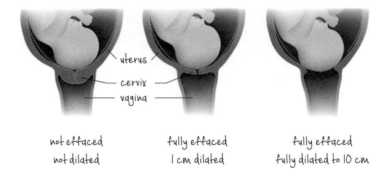

uterus
cervix
vagina

not effaced   fully effaced   fully effaced
not dilated   1 cm dilated   fully dilated to 10 cm

Sometimes labour is induced for the convenience of Mom or the doctor. In a healthy pregnancy you should not induce labour but rather let your baby determine when he is ready to be born. You may be advised to have labour induced if:

- you are past your due date and your baby's safety is a concern;
- you have medical issues such as preeclampsia that place you or your baby at risk;
- your baby is no longer growing adequately in utero.

If you want a natural delivery, induction for non-medical reasons should be avoided if possible.

Natural methods of induction

Your baby and the placenta are to a great extent responsible for the timing of labour, so natural methods of bringing on labour will only be successful if your baby is ready to be born. You can try a few safe and natural ways to get labour going, such as deep kissing, nipple stimulation and orgasm. This releases oxytocin, encouraging the start of labour at full term. Prostaglandins ripen the cervix sand are present in low quantities in semen – possibly not high enough to start labour, but making love won't do any harm.

Home remedies You may be told to try raspberry leaf tea and other herbal or homeopathic remedies and reflexology to induce labour naturally. However, there is no evidence-based information about whether they are effective.

Stretch and sweep If there is some ripening of the cervix (softening and shortened neck of the cervix), your doctor or midwife can stretch the cervix and sweep the membranes away from the lower uterine wall during a vaginal examination. This releases prostaglandins from the tissues and can help trigger labour. This is offered by midwives and obstetricians to reduce the need for medical induction and is felt to be safe.

Medical induction

Vaginal medications Ripening of the cervix can be achieved by introducing prostaglandins, usually vaginally, in the form of gel, tablets or an impregnated tape. Your doctor will predict the likelihood of successful induction by carefully assessing the cervix (its firmness, length, and how dilated it is, its orientation related to the vagina and the situation of your baby's head related to the pelvic inlet). This will guide the type and dosage of prostaglandins.

Catheter If introducing prostaglandins is not an option, labour may be induced using a catheter – a rubber tube with an inflatable balloon that is passed through the cervix and dilated once in place. This is rarely used anymore as prostaglandins are more effective

Artificial rupture of membranes Once the cervix is favourable, it might be possible to rupture the membranes (break the waters), which frequently initiates contractions.

Uterotonics are medication that cause the uterus to contract and are used to initiate contractions. Your pituitary gland releases oxytocin to stimulate contractions naturally. It is possible to administer synthetic oxytocin by intravenous drip to induce labour.

Disadvantages of induction

To induce is not a decision to take lightly, as it is associated with an increased need for pain relief, an increased occurrence of assisted delivery and an increased C-section rate, among other things. It is sometimes difficult to determine whether these outcomes are due to induction or related to the underlying cause of the need for induction.

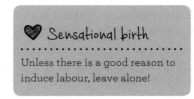

♡ Sensational birth
. . . .
Unless there is a good reason to
induce labour, leave alone!

   A possible side effect of induction is hyper-stimulating the uterus, which may place the foetus at risk. Therefore the decision must be appropriate, with the correct dosage, with monitoring.

Enema

Enemas should be used as a treatment for constipation, and not as a routine practice before or during birth. An enema is a liquid laxative squirted into your rectum to cause you to empty your bowel before birth. It is unnecessary.

IV line

A drip or intravenous line into your vein allows easy access for hydration and medication, and is required should you need an epidural, IV induction or C-section. It should not be necessary for a natural vaginal birth and is unpleasant as it interferes with your ability to change position, get in and out of the bath, to and from the toilet and to walk around during labour. It also makes it awkward to hold your baby when he's born. If you drink and eat in response to thirst and hunger during labour you shouldn't need additional electrolytes, glucose or hydration via an IV line.

Episiotomy

An episiotomy is a cut, made with surgical scissors, to enlarge the opening of the vagina. The cut is from the bottom of the vagina in a downwards direction, avoiding the anus, enabling the baby to pass through. Without an episiotomy there is a 30 to 60 per cent chance that the perineum will tear. A simple tear heals at least as well as a cut, so is often preferable.

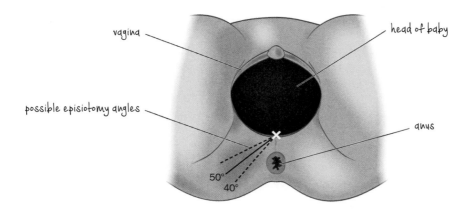

Episiotomy has been found to be more harmful than helpful in most circumstances and a recommended episiotomy rate is less than 20 per cent of vaginal births. An episiotomy is sometimes necessary to avoid a third degree tear (involving muscles) if there is a delay in delivering the head and some other emergency situation.

Forceps or vacuum

If delivery needs to be hastened during the second stage of labour (pushing), forceps or vacuum (ventouse) may be used to assist delivery. Assisted deliveries are performed by an obstetrician and can only be considered once you are fully dilated.

The choice of instrument will depend on specific circumstances as well as the preference and expertise of the obstetrician. Forceps have fallen out of favour because of an increased risk of trauma to Mom and Baby, and vacuum is more frequently performed.

- A ventouse is a cup-like instrument that attaches to the baby's head with suction (vacuum).
- Forceps are smooth, spoon-like instruments that are placed around the baby's head.

Assisted delivery is considered when there is concern over your baby's wellbeing or there is a delay in the second (pushing) stage as a result of:

- maternal fatigue;
- less than perfect position of your baby's head;
- having a large baby.

Assisted delivery is more common with epidural use and might require an episiotomy.

Other interventions

NATURAL GERMS

During vaginal delivery your baby will be exposed to bacteria and other germs that occur in your vagina and around the perineal area as he descends the birth canal and is born. While this may seem dirty to you, it has been found that these bacteria colonise your baby's gut and may be important in the development of good immunity, prevention of obesity, diabetes, allergies and asthma. So your baby receives his first inoculation in the miracle of a natural birth. This is yet another reason to choose natural delivery if you have the choice.

There is debate about the practice of placing a swab in the mother's vagina before C-section and wiping this across the baby's mouth after delivery. Further research is needed to ascertain if this provides similar protection to natural delivery and whether it is safe.

PLACENTAL ENCAPSULATION

The relatively recent practice of consuming your placenta is believed to have benefits such as increased energy, better mood, more breast milk, and prevention of postnatal depression. It is usually encapsulated – cleaned, steamed and dehydrated – before consumption.

Anecdotal evidence seems to be mostly positive, but there is no research that proves the claims. If you want to consume your placenta you need to arrange to have it kept for you, and it needs to be processed or frozen quickly or it will become rotten, like any other meat product.

STEM CELL STORAGE

The blood in your baby's placenta contains stem cells, which are the building blocks of our body's cells. They are primitive cells that have the ability to differentiate into all cell types. At present they can be used to treat cancers of the blood (leukaemia and lymphoma) and bone marrow failure. Research shows it is likely that stem cells might become a treatment for a much greater variety of illnesses, including diabetes and spinal cord injury.

Public stem cell banks are ideal where, with parental consent, stem cells are available to anyone who needs them. There are no public stem cell banks in South Africa yet.

It is now possible to capture these amazing stem cells from the placenta immediately after birth and store them for later use. In South Africa stem cells are stored in private banks and can be made available should your child or a sibling ever need them.

Deciding whether to bank your baby's stem cells is a big decision because it is very costly. There is also no guarantee that you will ever need to use them, so in a way, it's like an insurance policy – one you hope you won't need but, should the need arise, you may be grateful that you have it. It is possible that in the future new technologies will make cord stem cells redundant.

The correct collection method is vital to avoid contamination and to ensure that a large enough sample is collected.

The esSense of birth

- Your birth options lie on a continuum from very few interventions – as with a vaginal home-birth – through to the intervention of a C-section.

- A vaginal birth can be at home or in hospital and your baby may be delivered with you semi-reclining, upright or in a bath. It may be with or without the assistance of pain relief or interventions of induction, episiotomy, forceps or vacuum.

- A C-section may be done for medical reasons or simply because it is your choice. It may also be very unexpected. Accepting this route if it has not been planned very important for your emotional state.

- As you get more uncomfortable, you may start to consider inducing labour. It is important to know that this is an intervention that should be done for a medical reason rather than one of convenience.

- You can experience a sensational birth if you exercise your power to choose your ideal birth method and then release control, and accept that the process may not go completely according to this plan.

CHAPTER 15

Natural birth

At 40½ weeks Nontombi was more than ready for her labour to start. In the last week, she had hiked up to the Contour Path, eaten chilli at the Mexican Kitchen and had sex more often than in the whole of the last month, all in an attempt to initiate labour. Braxton Hicks contractions had been teasing her for the past three weeks and she was deliriously happy when she was woken at 3 am by strong contractions. She quietly tiptoed from their bed and climbed into a warm bath, waiting for these contractions to settle into a strong rhythm five minutes apart, which was when she planned to wake Thabo. By 7 am she was ready to go to hospital, where her obstetrician met her. Over the next four hours, she laboured in a bath and walking around, breathing through the contractions and managing to cope well with the pain. She was so relieved that the antenatal classes she had attended prepared her for this process. Not once did she feel out of control and she had a good sense of what to expect all along.

At 12:30, everything changed, the pain became unmanageable and she found herself begging for pain relief, but since she was 9 cm dilated, it was probably not worth an epidural. She panicked when the gas mask was offered and she put it over her nose and mouth, so she proceeded without any pain relief. One of the hardest parts of her second stage of labour was coordinating her pushes at the end. Bongani's head kept retreating into the birth canal after each push and Nontombi was tiring and feeling exhausted. Her obstetrician showed her the perineal area in a mirror and guided her hand to Bongani's head to feel how the contraction could help him emerge. Finally, at 1:40 pm, she delivered her perfect baby boy. This natural delivery was without question the hardest and yet the most ecstatic experience of Nontombi's life. Holding her warm wet baby boy and seeing the tears on Thabo's cheeks would be a memory indelibly etched in her mind. This is birth.

Labouring and giving birth is likely to be the most intense and awesome life experience, and no two births are the same. You will, like all mothers, have a sense of the birth you want, but you need to know that the most predictable aspect of birth is how unpredictable it is!

How you give birth matters and can be the most empowering and fulfilling experience of your life. Satisfaction is more often related to how you are treated during your baby's birth – with kindness, gentleness and respect, or lacking in these qualities – than the exact mode of delivery.

LABOUR

Labour is the process whereby your baby transitions from living in your uterus to being born. Imagine your baby is living in a room, opens a door, goes down a small passage and opens another door to get outside … that's it, simply put! The first door to open is the cervix, and this takes most of your labour time, the work being done by regular contractions of your uterus that push the baby down onto the cervix to slowly stretch and open it. The passage is the birth canal, and the second door is the perineum which stretches as you push with contractions once your cervix is fully open (10 cm dilated).

Cascade of hormones

There are a number of amazing hormones that initiate labour, help your uterus contract and your cervix soften, keep labour going and play a role in the transition of your baby to the world after birth:

Oxytocin, the love and attachment hormone, is also the ejection hormone. It peaks during male and female orgasm, causes contraction of the uterus and facilitates your milk ejection or letdown reflex – releasing milk from your breasts. In addition to causing contractions in labour, this hormone is responsible for the sense of euphoria you may experience in labour. Oxytocin is associated with intimacy, attachment and bonding and is transferred to your baby. It may protect him against the stresses of labour.

As oxytocin increases in labour, so do your contractions and this causes the painful lactic acid response in the muscles. As the pain increases, so your brain starts to release the next magic hormone – endorphins.

Endorphins are our naturally produced pain-relief hormones, mimicking the effects of opiates without negative side effects. They are painkillers and will make you feel a little calmer too, reducing the perception of pain. As you reach the end of your labour, it is common to feel heightened anxiety and even panic. This anxiety releases adrenaline, our flight, fight or fright hormone.

Adrenaline counters oxytocin, reducing oxytocin levels, which can slow down and interfere with labour in the first stage. This is why it's so very important that you feel safe and relaxed during labour. In the natural world, labour will stop in a mammal disturbed by a predator, and continue later when the animal feels safe again. Feeling safe during birth is important.

In the second stage of labour adrenaline can energise you for the final push. Adrenaline transfers to your baby in optimal levels, which helps him during labour and after birth. Having been exposed to adrenaline, babies born naturally are more alert in the first few hours after birth than those born by C-section.

Understanding how these hormones work can radically change the way your labour is managed:

- Labour progresses best when you feel safe and are in a familiar space where you feel comfortable. Privacy is also important.
- To speed up labour you may want to bring someone into the room, for instance a doula, who is relaxed and has a calming effect.
- A partner touching, massaging, distracting, using affirming words, kissing, stimulating your nipples, or just sitting quietly and supportively in the room can be beneficial in labour. Communicate what you are comfortable with.
- You may prefer to turn down the lights and encourage those around you to speak softly and gently and be calm.
- You may need someone to simply leave the room for you to feel safe again.

What causes pain in labour?

Intense uterine muscle contractions release lactic acid, which is that burning sensation you get when muscles are fatigued and working hard. The pressure of your baby's head on the cervix during a contraction stretches your cervix and that is experienced as a stretching pain behind your pubic bone. Your baby's head pressing down on your sacrum as he descends may give you backache owing to pressure on the lower back. It's important to remember that your contractions come and go regularly, and that you are in fact in pain for less time than you are *not* in pain. Use the periods between contractions to rest and recover before the next contraction comes.

How much pain you experience is very individual. Occasionally women don't experience pain in labour and, because they are waiting for it to get painful, don't even realise that they are in labour. Most women find labour hard work and intense, and managing their pain takes all of their attention and energy.

How you feel about the pain makes a big difference. If you are frightened and think that the pain means something is wrong, you will feel more tension and anxiety and will experience the pain as intense. You are more likely to find the pain manageable if you understand what is causing it. It is useful to picture your body opening up to allow your baby out in the way it is designed to, and capable of doing. The more relaxed and confident you feel about contractions, the better. It also helps if you are lucky enough to begin labour fresh, at the end of a rest, rather than the end of a long, tiring day.

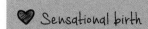

♥ Sensational birth
. . . .
About labour pain
· It is not continuous.
· It is manageable without medication.
· Labour is not fast and intense from start to finish.
· Crying and moaning is not a reaction to pain.
· Pain is not the enemy and not an indication that something is wrong.

Managing pain in labour: Natural, sensory pain relief

Natural pain-relief methods can be tried before you resort to medicated pain relief as they have no adverse side effects and enable your natural opiates, your endorphins, to act effectively.

The sensory world holds the secret to natural pain relief. Soothing sights and sounds combined with regulating touch and pressure are the secret to decreasing pain naturally in labour.

TOUCH AND PROPRIOCEPTION

Pain and temperature receptors travel along the same pathway (the anterolateral tract) to the brain and release hormones that alert the brain to danger. Proprioception from body position, pressure, and vibration and deep touch (massage) go along the dorsal column tract and result in the release of calming neurotransmitters. Knowing this can help you choose touch experiences that block the effect of pain.

Body position (proprioception) Your body position can give calming feedback. Stretching muscles and certain joint positions give wonderful feedback through the proprioceptive system.
- Moving, keeping upright, swaying, rocking and stretching the muscles come naturally in labour. As an added bonus, these movements help you to use gravity to position your baby for birth. They also keep you relaxed and less achy.
- Stretching tight, tense muscles between contractions is soothing – use yoga stretches and calf, hamstring and quad stretches. This can save you from cramping later on in labour.
- Sitting on the seat, facing the back, of an armless chair, gives you a lovely pelvic tilt and opens your legs, easing back pain.

You can lean on the back of the chair and easily get up after each contraction.

- Sitting on a Pilates ball is great for hip flexion and opening up your pelvis, as your legs are wide apart, but your weight is supported.
- Small bounces on the Pilates ball give wonderful soothing movement feedback too.

Massage Deep touch pressure is very calming and soothing, releases oxytocin and endorphins, and communicates love and care.

- Ask your birth partner to rub your lower back (sacral area). Direct palm pressure and circular firm massage are soothing for back pain during contractions. Massage shoulders between contractions to release tightness and tension.
- A foot massage is intimate yet unobtrusive. Having your partner touch the other end of your body between contractions brings pleasure and relaxation.
- Firm movement is mostly preferable to tickles, though large, feathery hands criss-crossed on your back can be pleasurable.

Temperature Neutral warmth close to body temperature or slightly higher is soothing for your whole body, while a lower temperature on your face and hands can be regulating.

- Being immersed in warm water is one of the best natural pain relievers – you are weightless in a bath, it's relaxing and distracting, and you feel safe and cocooned. Warm water has been shown to decrease pain and may speed up labour too.
- A warm shower is another option and you can even put a chair in the shower to sit on under the spray.
- Have a cool facecloth on hand to wipe your face after a tough contraction.

Vibration Like deep touch and proprioception, vibration releases calming neurotransmitters. Cats purr in labour and you can use your chest to create vibrations too.

- Pain, tension and fear lead to shallow breathing and sometimes breath-holding, which further increases pain and tension. Taking deep, slow breaths increases blood flow and relaxes your body. The rhythm of breathing in this manner takes you through the surge of pain so that you come to know that six or so breaths will get you to the other side of your contraction.

    The simplest method is slow in through your nose for four counts, and slow out for eight. Breathing out through your mouth, while relaxing your lower body, helps relax you where you need it most. Opening your mouth and relaxing your jaw has a similar effect on the cervix. You can also moan with each exhalation, which helps with this movement and elicits a soothing vibration sensation.
- The rhythmic repetition of contraction and relaxation can be used to create your own rituals for getting through each contraction. Focus on relaxing parts of your body, breathing slowly and moving in a rhythmic way, even dancing, rocking and moaning. All these things help to release tension and calm your body, so you can open nicely, and your baby can work his way down. In doing this, you are working with the contractions, rather than fighting against them.
- Laughter releases endorphins, so is a great pain-relief option. Smile and play a game like backgammon with your partner between contractions – the change of focus and laughter can help you relax.

SIGHT

Soothing visual input, similar to the womb world ,is calming.

Lighting Soft lighting makes you feel safe and at home, comfortable in the space, and also changes the way other people behave (more respectfully or reverently).

Visualisation You can influence the perception of pain simply by how you feel about your contractions. Pain usually invites a fear response, a sense that something is being hurt or damaged. This is not helpful in labour. You need to turn that around, knowing that this pain is a positive one, picturing how your cervix is opening with the stretching pain, like a flower unfolding and bursting open, or like a wave building up and crashing with the contraction. Visualising the positive effects of the pain can reduce it and will reduce your fear too.

SOUND

Soft, muted sounds, white noise and the sound of voices you know and love can help create a calming space, like in the womb.

- Choose music that calms you. Water sounds and music that you hear on a visit to the spa can be very soothing.
- Your own moans and humming may also soothe you.
- The sound of your partner's voice coaching you through a contraction with breathing techniques or giving you affirmation – how well you are doing – can be powerful in shifting your frame of mind in labour.
- On the other hand, you may find that you need silence to get through a contraction, and can communicate that to your partner.

SMELL

The sense of smell has direct links with the limbic part of the brain, where emotions and memories are stored. Use this powerful system to calm you or revive you when you are tiring. While you need to use essential oils in pregnancy with caution, you can use them in a diffuser or spray during labour for smells in the room. Do not add them to the bath water if your waters have broken.

- Lavender and black pepper have pain-relieving qualities. These can be used in massage oils in labour too.
- Frankincense is calming in the early stages of labour.
- Citrus, cloves and neroli are stimulating and may reduce anxiety (neroli) and decrease nausea (cloves).
- Flowers such as lavender and camomile are calming and create a sense of wellbeing.
- Using lovely smells also creates a new milieu and covers up clinical, foreign hospital smells.

Managing pain in labour: Medical pain relief

TRANSCUTANEOUS ELECTRICAL NERVE STIMULATION (TENS)

A TENS machine applies a low voltage electrical impulse through electrodes that attach to the skin in the areas supplied by specific nerve roots in the lower back. This impulse seems to control pain signals and help release endorphins. It's hired for the weeks leading up to the birth and should be used daily before labour so you are familiar with its use. It can help to relieve backache, help you sleep better before your labour starts, and help manage pain during labour.

Benefits It can be applied and controlled by you and can be used outside a hospital setting.

Disadvantages It can't be used if you are in water. Some women find it distracting trying to manage their TENS machine while labouring. There is some uncertainty as to whether the effect of TENS is any more than placebo.

Entonox, gas and air or 'laughing gas'
This is a mixture of 50 per cent nitrous oxide in oxygen, which is breathed in through a mouthpiece. It is calming and can take the edge off the pain.

Benefits It is easy to use and self-administered. The onset of action is within 20 to 30 seconds, and the effect wears off quickly. Entonox is a useful analgesic for the transition stage or while waiting for an epidural.

Disadvantages It can cause drowsiness and sometimes nausea. It causes a dry mouth.

Painkillers
Pethidine and morphine are in a class of painkillers called opiates and are usually given by injection (into the muscle or occasionally intravenously).

Benefits Opiates are powerful painkillers, reducing the intensity of pain, although not removing the sensation of pain completely. Where epidurals are not available they do provide relief.

Disadvantages Opiates will make you drowsy and frequently cause nausea, so they should always be given with medication to prevent nausea.

These painkillers cross the placenta and, if given late in labour, can make your baby less attentive, sleepier and less able to establish breast-feeding. This can be counteracted with an antidote injection. In overdose, opiates will suppress respiration in the mother – they must be given in the correct dose. For all these reasons they are not an ideal painkiller in active labour.

Epidural
An epidural is a form of regional anaesthesia – local anaesthetic is administered to the nerve roots that supply the abdomen and lower body as they leave the spinal cord. This temporarily blocks the sensation of pain (and temperature, which is detected by the same nerve fibres). The sensation of touch and pressure and the ability to move muscles are less affected, depending on the dose.

Your anaesthetist will insert a cannula (a thin tube) through a needle to lie just outside the membranes surrounding the spinal cord. This remains in place until after delivery, so the amount of pain relief can be adjusted.

Benefit An epidural is very safe and are the most effective form of pain relief. Once it is working you won't be aware of pain at all. As well as providing pain relief, it also allows you to relax and rest. High adrenaline and pain levels can cause ineffective contractions

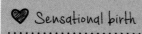

♥ Sensational birth

Epidural
If you choose to have an epidural, you will know when the time is right, as you will feel the pain intensify to a point that feels unmanageable for you. Remember that it takes time for the anaesthetist to arrive and set up the epidural.

and labour may progress better with an epidural. An epidural will lower your blood pressure, an advantage in patients with high blood pressure.

Your power for pushing is not reduced by an epidural.

Disadvantages You will need an intravenous drip when having an epidural, so that you can be given fluids to counteract an abnormal drop in blood pressure. Because you will be unaware of your bladder filling, a catheter will be inserted after the epidural has taken to keep your bladder empty. Your baby's heart rate will be monitored electronically. You will probably not be able to get up and walk around.

The second stage of labour (birth itself) is longer with an epidural. Your sensation of the urge to push is absent with an epidural and this can indirectly reduce the efficiency of pushing. As long as you and your baby are well, more time is allowed for the second stage of labour. It is also useful to reduce the intensity of the epidural once you are fully dilated so that you will feel some urge to push.

There is an increased chance of an assisted delivery (forceps or vacuum) with an epidural.

Although it is the safest form of anaesthesia, there are side effects and complications that you need to be aware of, ranging from the more common nausea to headaches, which are rare. Your doctor should discuss these with you should you choose to have an epidural.

Spinal block

Spinal block is similar to an epidural, except that the local anaesthetic is injected into the cerebrospinal fluid (CSF), which bathes the spinal cord.

The needle is inserted between the vertebrae and through the membranes (the dura) surrounding the spinal cord. The local anaesthetic is administered as a once-off injection – no cannula is left in place.

Benefits Compared with an epidural, a spinal block takes effect faster and the pain relief occurs sooner (almost immediately). The pain relief can be more effective.

Disadvantages The effect lasts between three and seven hours. While this is more than enough time for a C-section, it might not last long enough to get you through labour.

How do I know I'm in labour?

As your body prepares for labour, your cervix (the tightly closed opening of the uterus) softens, tilts forward (from posterior to anterior position) and shortens (effaces). The mucous plug in the cervix, which protects your baby from infection during pregnancy, falls way. You will know this has happened when you have a bloody mucous discharge, which may or may not have some brown or even fresh blood in it. This is called a **show** and may occur a day or so before labour starts.

Your labour may begin with regular uterine contractions or rupture of membranes (waters breaking). If your membranes rupture without regular contractions beginning within a few hours, you should contact your caregiver to manage the next step.

Labour overview

Each labour is so very different. Labour contractions usually start far apart (10 to 20 minutes), and last as short as 20 seconds; this is a mild contraction. With time, they increase in intensity and duration, and become closer together; a moderate contraction lasts 20 to 40 seconds. The contractions of active labour usually last 40 to 60 seconds (a strong contraction), and are 3 to 5 minutes apart.

FOUR STAGES OF LABOUR

In giving birth, you will pass through four stages of labour:
- 1st stage: Early through active labour to transition phase – dilate 0–10 cm
- 2nd stage: Birth – fully dilated to birthing your baby
- 3rd stage: Delivering the placenta
- 4th stage: Recovery

This is when you should be heading to hospital, or calling your midwife.

The effect of your uterus tightening is to push your baby down so that his head is pressing firmly onto your cervix, stretching and opening it, until it is fully dilated.

Once the cervix is fully dilated, your baby can emerge from the uterus and descend through the birth canal. At this point you will get a strong urge to push, as if you were defecating. Thereafter you will bear down or push with each contraction. Your perineum will stretch a little more with each push, until your baby's head, and then his body, can fit through the birth canal.

First stage: Early labour

Early labour (latent labour), from the start of your regular contractions until active labour (3 strong contractions in 10 minutes) can take a couple of hours to a couple of days, but averages at 3 to 12 hours long.

What's happening?
- Your cervix will dilate from 0–4 cm.
- Your contractions will last 20 to 60 seconds.
- They will start 20 minutes apart, becoming more frequent, longer and more intense. Towards the end of this stage they will be 5 minutes apart.
- You will be able to hold a conversation during a contraction and will probably cope well at home.
- Your partner can:
  » help you relax;
  » help you to breathe when the contractions start to get tough;
  » remind you to empty your bladder;
  » time the contractions.

What to do in early labour
You may be feeling terribly excited and also quite apprehensive, just like you feel before running your first half-marathon or starting an event you've trained for but don't know quite how you're going to manage. In much the same way, pace yourself, rest and relax when you can, allowing the cycle of contraction and relaxing of your uterus to get into a rhythm. If you can have a conversation while your uterus contracts, you are likely still to be in the early labour phase.

Get up and move about – go for a walk. Drink when thirsty and eat small high-energy snacks, like fruit, energy bars, nuts and biltong if you feel hungry. Empty your bladder every hour or when it feels a bit full.

First stage: Active labour

Active labour takes place from when your cervix is 4 cm dilated and you are having three strong contractions every 10 minutes until you are ready to push (fully dilated).

What's happening?
- Your cervix will dilate from 4–8 cm.
- Your contractions will be 40 to 90 seconds long.

- They will be 2 to 4 minutes apart.
- This stage can take from 3 to 8 hours.
- You will need to concentrate through each contraction and the pain may be intense.
- Your partner can:
  » help you concentrate;
  » help you to breathe when the contractions start to get tough;
  » massage your lower back or feet;
  » offer drinks and snacks between contractions;
  » encourage and affirm you.

WHAT TO DO IN ACTIVE LABOUR

Your contractions are coming close together and are more intense. If you have set up a good ritual in early labour with positions to labour in, relaxation techniques to enable you to rest between contractions and your support person working with you, you will enter this phase with some confidence. If you are birthing in hospital you will head there once you are having 3 strong contractions in 10 minutes. When admitted to hospital you will need to settle into your new space and make it your own, finding your rhythm again.

Transition

As your body transitions from labour to birthing your baby, you may feel a little panicky. It may reassure you to know you are likely to be close to the end.

WHAT'S HAPPENING?

- You will dilate from 8–10 cm.
- Your contractions will be 60 to 90 seconds long.
- They will be 60 to 90 seconds apart and you may feel like there is too little recovery time.
- This stage can take between 30 minutes and 3 hours.
- Your partner can:
  » stay with you – it's not a time to be alone;
  » help you to focus your breathing until fully dilated;
  » suggest a more comfortable position;
  » affirm you and help you to stay calm;
  » wipe your face with a cool cloth and offer you sips of water between contractions.

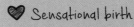

♥ Sensational birth

You are unique
Every birth is unique and this description is a guideline only. Your caregiver will guide your labour.

WHAT TO DO IN TRANSITION

Just before your cervix becomes fully dilated your labour may change and your contractions may become very intense, a point at which many women who have been managing well become overwhelmed, and feel like they can't go on. It may be too late for an epidural if birth is felt to be imminent and this is when a confident birth partner, doula or midwife can help you to keep focus and regain calm. You are almost at the last straight – the end is in sight! Some transitions involve a resting period of 10 to 15 minutes, when the uterus appears to gear up for the final lap.

Second stage of labour: Birth

This is the time that you will push actively with contractions to birth your baby.

What's happening?

- You are fully dilated and feel an uncomfortable urge to push or bear down during contractions.
- Your contractions will be 40 to 75 seconds long.
- They will be 3 to 5 minutes apart.
- This stage can take between 10 minutes and 2 hours.
- Your partner can:
  - » encourage you and tell you of progress made;
  - » offer you sips of water if you are thirsty.

When to push

When you feel the urge to bear down it feels the same as when you urgently need to poo. This means that your cervix is completely dilated and your baby's head has moved down, which signals the exciting last lap before meeting your baby.

The stretching in your cervix during contractions in active labour changes to the stretching of your perineum as you bear down during the contractions. If you have had an epidural and don't have the urge to push with contractions, you should be allowed to wait a while for the epidural to wear off so that you feel the urge to push when you have contractions. There is usually no rush to push immediately.

Pushing or bearing down comes naturally. Take a deep breath and push as you breathe out, or hold your breath as you push. You don't need to be told when or how to push; it's best to listen to and follow your own body. You will probably manage about 3 to 4 pushes with each contraction, the baby's head emerging a little more with each push and then subsiding back inside as the contraction fades and you rest until the next one. It is normal to push for 30 minutes to 2 hours. This allows the perineum time to stretch and shouldn't be unnecessarily rushed. If the pushing is not successful and there is some urgency to deliver your baby, delivery is assisted with forceps or vacuum to help ease your baby out as you push.

Your baby's birth

When the widest part of the baby's head is at the perineum this is called **crowning**. It feels extremely intense and you will feel compelled to push your baby out, using all your strength. As your baby's head slides out, you will feel huge relief, and your caregiver will feel at his neck for the cord. If it is wrapped around his neck it can be looped over his head, or if too tight to do this, it will be clamped on either side and cut between the two clamps.

If there is evidence of meconium in your amniotic fluid, your baby's mouth and nose will be suctioned so that meconium doesn't get inhaled when he breathes for the first time.

There is often a pause before the next contraction, allowing the baby to turn slightly so that the shoulders can move into position for the final push. When you next push, the shoulders are released and the rest of your baby slips out. Your baby can be delivered onto your tummy, with the cord still attached, and dried and welcomed. A well baby should be pink, breathing, possibly crying, and curled up in a foetal position, not limp and floppy.

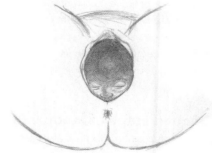

CORD CLAMPING AND CUTTING

The umbilical cord has provided nutrients and oxygen and removed carbon dioxide and waste for the duration of pregnancy. Once your baby has been born and taken his first breath, this is no longer required. Exposure to air, with its different temperature and atmospheric pressure, causes the vessels of the cord to go into spasm and it will naturally stop pulsating after a few minutes.

Traditionally your baby's cord will be clamped and cut once he is born. Once the cord has been cut, a little of the cord blood (which is foetal blood) is collected for a thyroid test. In the case of a mother whose blood type is rhesus negative, the sample will also be used to determine the baby's blood group.

Delaying cord clamping

For the first few minutes after birth, blood in the cord and placenta is still transferred to your baby. This is beneficial for your baby, increasing the amount of blood he has and reducing the chance of anaemia, especially in premature or low birth-weight babies. For this reason, it is often recommended that you **delay cord clamping** for at least one minute or until it has stopped pulsating. Do not worry if this is not possible – the benefit is less important in a healthy, mature baby.

Third stage of labour

While you are welcoming your baby, powerful uterine contractions reduce the maternal blood flow to the placenta and cause it to shear off and come away. This takes 5 to 30 minutes and then it is expelled via the vagina. Your caregiver might ask you to cough or push gently to expel the placenta. An injection of oxytocin into your thigh is recommended to assist with the expulsion of the placenta and to reduce the risk of post-partum haemorrhage. You will hardly notice either the injection or expelling the placenta, as you are so captivated by your baby.

If there was a tear or cut requiring stitches this will be done soon after the placenta is out, with local anaesthetic to numb the area needing stitches.

Surprises around birth

- Nausea and even vomiting in labour are not uncommon – don't be alarmed. They are often a sign that the labour is in the transition phase and birth is fast approaching or may simply be an indication of the intensity of the pain. If you've eaten a fair meal recently, they could be a result of your digestion halting during labour.
- When your epidural is started, the resulting drop in blood pressure can make you nauseous. Pain medication can also make you nauseous.
- Getting the shakes after the baby is born happens due to the change in hormones and the endorphin release. Anaesthetic given during a spinal block for a C-section can also leave you shaking. Placing heavy blankets on you or rubbing your legs can help with this.
- To decrease the bleeding from the placental site, your midwife or obstetrician will place a hand on your abdomen, at around your belly button, and massage your uterus to make it contract.
- Passing a stool is normal and common when you are bearing down, so don't feel inhibited or shy. Chances are that you won't even notice, and it is easily wiped away and disposed of.

Healthy birth practices

With a view to having a natural birth with less chance of intervention (if this is your birth preference), note the following:

- Let labour begin on its own – your baby actually initiates labour when he is ready to be born.
- Unless medically necessary, avoid interventions. Your baby's heart rate must be monitored, but continuous foetal monitoring (which limits your movement and position in labour) is not necessary. Eating or drinking restrictions, episiotomies, IV fluids, epidural, artificial rupture of the membranes and oxytocin augmentation are not necessary for uncomplicated labour.
- Walk and move around, keeping active during labour. This helps enormously with pain relief and eases your baby into the best birth position.
- Bring a loved one, friend or doula for support. This is likely to make you feel safer, therefore more relaxed, and also encouraged and supported.
- Avoid birthing flat on your back, as blood flow to the baby may be inhibited, and you are effectively pushing uphill in this position. Let gravity help you.
- Follow your natural urge to push, as this usually is the most effective way to birth your baby.
- Take your birth plan to the labour room to communicate your wishes and hopes to your caregivers so that they are more likely to be realised.

BECOMING A MOM

Your baby begins his life as part of you, an egg that you have carried for your entire life until the moment of conception. In that moment, a new person, an independent soul, begins to form. And with that begins the paradox of motherhood.

A part of you that has been 100 per cent dependent and within you has to become independent and separate and exist apart from you. And it is your role to facilitate this transition from dependence to independence. It is a "push-pull dance of connection and separation, independence and dependence"

♡ Sensational birth

Ingredients for a sensational birth:
- Know your birth preferences.
- Trust your body – you are powerful.
- Choose the right labour assistance – partner and/ or doula or midwife.
- Don't rush to hospital in early labour – labour takes time.
- Create a sensory soothing birth space.

- Keep moving through labour.
- Be open to changes of plans and know your options and preferences.
- Be positive and calm – breathing and meditation will help.
- Cuddle your baby skin to skin after birth.

(Ann Pleshette Murphy – *The Seven Stages of Motherhood*). This dance will preoccupy every day of motherhood – the overwhelming feeling to hold and contain and protect your baby will be challenged by the knowledge that each day you will and must facilitate his independence and separation from you.

That first separation, the first enormous transition from dependence to independence, happens with birth. For nine months there is no separation and there is full dependence, and in the moment of the umbilical cord cutting you enter a journey towards being separate. You will be overcome and bereft in the same moment as elated and filled with joy. This is birth.

The esSense of natural birth

- Oxytocin, endorphins and adrenaline are the hormones of labour.

- The pains of labour and delivery are produced by the profound changes within your body of your uterus contracting, the cervix dilating and the vagina and perineum stretching. This pain is not continuous but comes in waves, with periods between contractions that are pain free.

- Natural pain management centres on using the sensory system to manage the sensations. Visualisation and the way you think about pain can help to control your response to the contractions. There are no adverse effects to these methods.

- Medical pain relief includes gas, opiates and epidural. Each of these interventions has positives and negatives.

- There are four stages in labour, the first being the longest as you dilate. The second stage is birth itself, which lasts 20 minutes to 2 hours. The third stage involves birthing the placenta. The final stage is recovery.

CHAPTER 16

Out of your hands

Sandy had never imagined she would be bent over an incubator in the NICU, staring at a tiny human being who was hooked up to tubes and lines, instead of cuddling and nurturing a perfect newborn. It was breaking her heart that she could hardly hold Chelsea and she felt completely ill-equipped for this situation.

The nightmare started when Sandy's waters broke at 34 weeks. She had been on bed rest for a week at around 30 weeks and then, when everything seemed okay, she found herself in hospital, preparing for the birth of her baby six weeks early. She had been given steroid injections and now was facing a situation she was simply not prepared for.

Pregnancy is an adjustment, even when things go well. When plans change and your pregnancy and baby become medical territory, it can make you feel very out of control and anxious.

PREMATURE LABOUR

If you go into labour before 37 completed weeks of pregnancy, it is considered premature. Premature birth puts your baby at risk for complications, especially if your little one is born before 34 weeks. For this reason, every effort will be made to keep your baby *in utero*, if medically possible.

Managing premature labour involves:

- recognising labour;
- making sure there are no risks to stopping labour;
- attempting to stop it;
- preparing your baby for premature birth.

Stopping labour

If there are risks to continued pregnancy, for example if you have an intrauterine infection, your baby is in distress or your placenta separates from the uterus, premature delivery is better than ongoing pregnancy. In almost all other cases, your baby will be better off in the uterus than in the most highly specialised neonatal intensive care unit (NICU). For this reason you may receive medication to stop the uterine contractions.

By stopping labour, your doctor will buy time (48 hours) to give you injections of corticosteroids (cortisone). This helps your baby's lungs to mature and significantly improves the outcome for your baby if she is born early. This time can also be used to transfer you to a hospital with NICU facilities. Having steroid injections is safe and an essential component of managing premature labour. The cortisone is given as two injections, once daily on two consecutive days.

BED REST

You will be hospitalised for treatment if you are in premature labour and will remain in hospital if the threat of delivery is imminent. Bed rest or reduced activity may be recommended. There is little evidence that bed rest does any good; it may in fact cause more problems. You will be advised what is appropriate in your case.

Premature delivery

Should early delivery be necessary, it needs to be at a facility with NICU care. The type of delivery will be determined by the degree of prematurity – very premature babies are best delivered by C-section to avoid distress and trauma. Continuous electronic foetal monitoring is usually recommended.

If your baby is born before 34 weeks, a paediatrician will be present at delivery and your baby will be admitted to and cared for in an NICU. After 34 weeks, this will depend on your baby's condition.

Unless she needs immediate resuscitation, delayed cord clamping (see p. 141) is beneficial for your premature baby.

ADJUSTING YOUR DREAM

During pregnancy you begin the process of bonding with your little one. You envisage your baby, who she will be and what she will look like. You have a picture of your birth and the way in which you will meet this precious person. When your baby is born prematurely, the reality will not match your dream.

The premature birth of a baby will evoke different emotions in different people. Some parents may feel anger or sadness, while others may experience denial and be detached or emotionally removed from the situation. Whatever your response, you will be faced with a period of adjustment.

You may grieve for the loss of your dream birth and perfectly healthy newborn. If your baby is very ill, you may fear that she may die or be disabled. When contemplating the worst-case scenario, you may be preparing to grieve the loss of a healthy baby. Another very strong emotion, especially for Mom, is guilt. You may feel that you have not been an adequate incubator for your baby or have not met your own expectations of delivering a healthy baby.

If you want more information on your premature baby's care in the NICU, read *Prematurity – Adjusting your dream* by Welma Lubbe (Little Steps, 2008).

BEING AN ACTIVE PARENT IN THE NEONATAL UNIT

You may initially feel daunted and at the mercy of the staff in the neonatal unit but will soon recognise your central role in the care of your baby. As the most consistent caregiver and the only member of the team who cannot be replaced, you are in a position to meet your baby's needs:

- **You are the consistent caregiver.** You are the most consistent person around your baby. Staff will come and go and change shifts but you are a constant in your child's life. With time you will be the one who knows your baby's signals and whom she perceives as consistent and predictable on a sensory level.
- **Speak for your baby.** You will observe her responses to interventions and you will know what sensory input she needs.
- **Understand her state.** Your baby has a unique language that will tell you whether she is coping well or distressed. Get to know her signals so that you can interpret her responses and her ability to tolerate an interaction at a specific time.

Your premature baby's state and signals

Like any full-term baby, your premature baby can be in deep sleep, light sleep, a drowsy state, calm alert state or active alert state, or she can be distressed and crying.

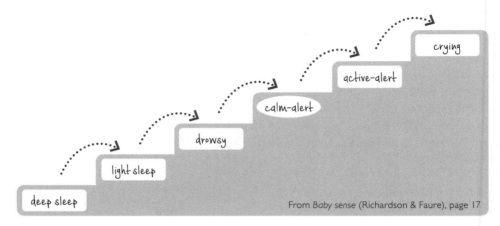

From *Baby sense* (Richardson & Faure), page 17

- **Deep sleep** is essential for your premature baby's growth and in this state she will sleep through most noises and sensory stimulation in the neonatal unit. If she is in a very deep sleep state, try not to disturb her with painful interventions as this is a vital time for her growth and development.
- **Light sleep** is the state in which your premature baby will spend much of her day. She is processing the interventions and interactions of the day and is easily woken. While in light sleep, she may give you 'back off' signals, such as splaying of fingers and saluting.
- When in a **drowsy** state your baby opens and closes her eyes and is responsive to the world. She takes her time in responding and is not learning much from her world but is awake.
- In the **calm alert** state, your baby is breathing smoothly and is settled and may engage with you for brief periods. Before 32 weeks, your baby will spend almost no time in this state and therefore should not be stimulated. You will need to watch carefully for her signals. Periods in the calm alert state get longer as your baby gets older and you will be able to engage with her for longer periods of time.
- **Active alert** is the state in which your premature baby is having a hard time self-regulating and is no longer enjoying interaction. Just a small amount of stimulation or interaction is enough to push a premature baby into overstimulation and the active alert state. In this state, she will be trying to settle herself or protect herself from interventions.
- The **crying** state is distressing for your premature baby and uses energy she needs for growth and healing. She will experience irregular breathing and her oxygen levels may drop. Crying is a stress signal that tells you your baby has had enough. You need to help her to calm down and regulate her state.

The states you most want to encourage are the content deep or light sleep states and the calm alert state. In these states your premature baby grows, has optimal oxygenation levels and begins to interact.

Signs that I'm coping: When your baby is showing signs of coping, she is in the calm alert state. This is the time to engage and interact with her:
- She is awake and calm.
- Her heart rate and breathing are stable and regular.

- She has limited body movements.
- She looks at you and may focus on your face.
- She is pink and her oxygen saturation levels are good.

Signs that I'm trying to cope: Signs that your baby is trying to cope show that she is reaching a level of stress and is attempting to self-regulate. These are healthy signals and show that your premature baby is growing up:
- Non–nutritive sucking
- Putting her hands near her face
- Placing her hands under her chin
- Grasping your finger

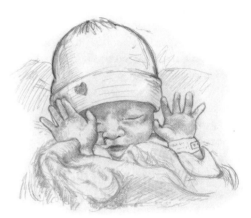

Signs that I'm stressed: If you see the following signals, communicate with her team so that an intervention can be paused if she is becoming more stressed:
- She may arch her back, stretch out her arms and legs and splay her fingers.
- Her heart rate is too low or too high and her oxygenation levels decrease.
- She may frown, yawn, hiccup or sneeze.
- Your baby may become blue around the mouth as her breathing changes.
- She may move frantically or look away trying to escape the stimuli.

SENSORY CARE IN THE NEONATAL UNIT

The womb is a perfect sensory world for your baby's development. The critical interventions that will save your baby's life in the neonatal unit may be difficult for her to tolerate on a sensory level. Since the sensory environment of the neonatal unit can put your baby's long-term development at risk, sensory developmental care is used in many neonatal units across the world.

Follow these guidelines:
- When your baby is still medically fragile, her medical needs may take precedence over sensory developmental care.
- Ask the medical team when it is reasonable to put in place sensory care for your premature baby.
- Follow the principles of the womb for ideas on sensory developmental care.

Touch

The touch system is well developed at birth and is sensitive. *In utero* touch is containing and positive as opposed to the many negative touch experiences a

> ★ Sense-able secret
>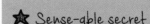
> When premature babies are closely monitored to prevent sensory overload, they have a better developmental outcome for at least 36 months, are weaned faster from the respirator and tube feedings, and have a lower incidence of haemorrhaging and chronic lung disease, a shorter hospital stay and lower cost.

baby has to endure in the neonatal unit. Use positive touch to counteract the unpleasant experiences of the neonatal unit.

- **Deep, still touch** helps your premature baby feel contained, much like the constant touch of the womb walls. Place both of your warmed hands open over your baby's body using firm pressure. She may take a few seconds to adjust to the touch. Do not move your hands; relax your shoulders and keep the pressure deep as opposed to light touch which is disconcerting. Within a short time you will feel your baby relax and her breathing stabilise. You can use this strategy after painful interventions and to help her settle.
- Use rolled blankets or special positioning aids to contain her – to create **boundaries** for your premature baby to move up against. A boundary around her head is particularly soothing for her as it creates a sense of containment similar to the womb.
- Offer your finger for your baby to grasp onto if she splays her fingers.
- **Kangaroo care** is very beneficial for your baby. Place your premature baby, with only a nappy and a hat on, on your bare chest. Cover her with a blanket or wear a kangaroo care top. Your chest temperature will rise a degree or two to warm your baby up and remain constant. Do this **as often as possible** as soon as your team gives the go-ahead – usually once she is relatively stable.
- Maintain a **constant temperature** in the incubator or in kangaroo care.
- **Cluster** painful interventions so that your premature baby can have periods of undisturbed sleep as often as possible. If the intervention becomes too much for her and she is distressed, give her a time-out by stopping the intervention and giving deep, still touch, unless her medical needs override this.
- **Sucking** on a dummy is soothing non-nutritive sucking. During stressful or painful procedures, give your baby a premature baby dummy to suck on. In addition to soothing her, this will facilitate maturation of the sucking reflex.
- **Swaddle** her when she is being removed from the incubator and, as she gets older, swaddle her in the incubator too. She should be swaddled with her legs slightly bent towards her tummy and with her hands together near her face.

> **BENEFITS OF KANGAROO CARE**
> - Better weight gain as less energy is used to maintain a calm state and a constant temperature
> - Encourages breast-feeding earlier
> - Stable heart rate and breathing and therefore good oxygen saturation levels
> - Reduced hospital infections
> - Earlier discharge and therefore lower hospital costs
> - Positive feelings for Mom and Baby promote bonding

Vision

Your baby's visual system is the least developed sense and needs to be almost entirely protected until she is at full-term age or discharged:

- Dim the lights of the entire neonatal unit and rather use direct lighting over only the incubator when medical procedures or general care is being carried out.
- When the bright lights need to be switched on for procedures, cover your premature baby's eyes.
- If your baby is in a closed incubator, you can place a towel or blanket on top of the incubator to dim the light further and protect her eyes.

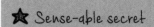
Sense-able secret

Try to carry out interventions with two caregivers – one to do the medical or caregiving intervention and the other to watch the baby's signals and help her self calm.

- The light in the neonatal unit can cycle, simulating day and night – brighter lighting in the day and dimmer at night.

Sound

At times you may have difficulty controlling sounds in the neonatal unit. Make a mental note to listen for any sound that is louder than a gentle voice.

- Talk to your team about decreasing the levels of the alarms and respond quickly to them.
- Turn your mobile phone onto vibrate as the jarring sound of a ringing mobile phone is very unsettling.
- Do not place anything on the roof of a closed incubator as the sound is magnified inside the incubator.
- Close doors of cabinets and the portholes of the incubator very quietly.
- If your baby's incubator is near an area of high traffic, ask that she be moved to a quieter space.
- Turn off radios or limit usage to soft music.
- Play a white noise CD or app gently in the background to mask the jarring sounds of the neonatal unit.

Movement and gravity

Sensory care for the vestibular and postural system is important for your baby's motor development later.

- Positioning is very important for your premature baby. Since the pull of gravity has a big effect on your baby's low muscle tone, you need to put your baby in a position as close as possible to the contained, curled-up position of the womb.
- Position your baby in a curled-up position, preferably on her side. On her side, her arms are brought together and close to her face, making her feel more contained. Place the boundary or nest around her head, down her back and around her legs to tuck them towards her chest.
- If your baby is lying on her back, support her head on a gel or memory foam mattress or pillow to prevent flattening of her head; her head should be in line with her spine. Use a boundary or nest to support her legs and shoulders so that she is slightly curled up and not flat on her back in a frog-like pose.
- Placing your premature baby on her tummy in the neonatal unit is a very good idea. This is a good position for breathing, absorbing feeds, development and feeling secure. Since her breathing is monitored, there is no risk of SIDS in this position. When she is on her tummy, place a roll of fabric that is narrower than her shoulders under her tummy and chest. It should run from her belly button under her chest and head. This will encourage her shoulders to come forward and create a flexed shape – not flattening of her chest. Her knees should be tucked under her tummy.

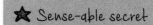

★ Sense-able secret

Be cautious when using disposable nappies with your premature baby. Premature babies have less collagen (strengthening fibres) in their skin, making it vulnerable to forming blisters and skin damage if the adhesive tape on disposable nappies sticks to the skin.

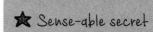

★ Sense-able secret

The optimal position for your baby to grow, develop and stay calm is:
· Curled towards the belly button, except her neck which is straight
· Shoulders rounded forward
· Hands near mouth
· Knees together

Smell and taste

Your baby's sense of smell is so sensitive and will be affected in the neonatal unit.

- Limit the number of invasive procedures involving her mouth, such as changing tubes and suctioning. Keep them to the bare minimum needed for her survival and cluster them.
- Don't open alcohol swabs, which smell very strong, or use strong-smelling cleaning agents near your baby's face.
- Kangaroo care or skin-to-skin contact allows your baby to be contained near the soothing smell of Mom or Dad.
- If your baby is having a nasogastric (NG) feed, combine this with kangaroo care so she associates your smell and touch contact with the soothing feeling of a full tummy.
- Do not wear perfume or aftershave at all when visiting your baby and be aware of the smell of detergent on your clothes.

FEEDING YOUR PREMATURE BABY

Your premature baby needs to be feeding well before she will be discharged. The road to feeding your premature baby effectively starts early.

Early feeds

If your baby is ill or born very early, she may be given essential hydration and nutrients via nasogastric tube or even a drip in the early days. In time the NG tube will be used to feed her breast milk or formula until she can suck.

Encouraging sucking

The sucking reflex needs to be established and encouraged with non-nutritive sucking. Your baby can suck a prem baby dummy, your clean finger or her thumb. Offering your emptied (expressed) breast will help her develop the coordination of sucking without having to cope with coordinating swallowing milk and breathing too. Offer non-nutritive sucking while she is feeding from an NG tube and after a feed, and also when she is distressed and for at least 10 minutes a day when she is in the drowsy or awake states.

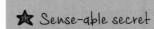

★ Sense-able secret

The benefits of non-nutritive sucking:

- It is soothing and helps your baby to regulate her state and stay in the calm alert state.
- It prepares her for feeding.
- She can practise how to coordinate suck, swallow and breathe.
- It assists with digestion.

Expressing

Express your first breast milk as soon as possible after the birth of your baby (preferably within an hour to four hours). Colostrum and early milk is particularly enriched with calories and antibodies. Although it may be some time before your baby can drink your expressed breast milk, you can freeze the milk for when she can tolerate milk in a tube feed or bottle.

Keep these tips in mind:

- Have a lactation consultant to assist you.
- Before expressing apply warmth (heated wet towels or a happy hugger) and massage your breast to release colostrum.
- Initially expect a few drops to a teaspoon or two.

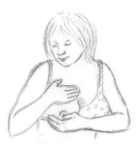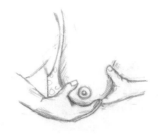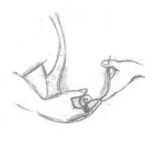

- Hand expressing, if you have the knack, is the most effective way of extracting your milk until more volume comes in on day 3 or 4. If there is no one to help you hand express comfortably then pump two to four-hourly.
- Using a double electric breast pump works most efficiently.
- Express from each breast for 5 to 10 minutes every 2 to 4 hours until your milk comes in.
- Once your milk comes in, continue to express until the breast milk flow slows right down, after roughly 10 to 15 minutes per side.
- You shouldn't need to express for more than 30 minutes at a time, if you are single pumping, or 15 to 20 minutes if you are double pumping. Breast compression while pumping increases the volume expressed.
- Limit wake ups during the night to express – you need your rest. Pump before going to sleep and once between 2 and 4 am and again on waking.
- It's important not to exceed six-hour stretches between emptying your breasts in the first six weeks, as you are establishing your milk supply.
- Try to express with a picture of your baby in front of you or where you can see her; this will help with the release of let-down hormones.
- After a week or so of expressing, you will find you can express much more milk in each sitting.
- Most women need to express seven times a day to produce a full milk supply, which adds up to three-hourly between 7 am and 7 pm, plus two expressings between 7 pm and 7 am.

Cup feeds

If your baby is not ready to start breast-feeding you may offer milk to her in a cup (you can use the sterilised cap of a bottle). Place the cup or cap near her lips so that she learns to lap the milk, much like a kitten.

Breast- or bottle-feeds

Once your baby can coordinate swallowing and breathing while sucking and can maintain an awake state, she will be ready to start having breast feeds. Many premature babies only manage this after 34 weeks.

Breast milk is essential for premature babies as it protects their digestive tract in a way that formula cannot. Bottle-feeding expressed milk can be avoided if good lactation support is available. Breast milk from a breast-milk bank is preferable to formula if you cannot express.

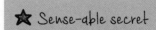

☆ Sense-able secret

It is important to note that premature babies have lower tolerance levels for stimuli and that they should be treated with extra care with regard to sensory input, especially at feeding time.

Is my baby ready to feed?

It is important to wait until your baby is ready to start feeding by sucking. Your team will guide you on when to start but here are a few guidelines:

- Your baby must be medically well and stable.
- Her heart rate and breathing will be regular and stable.
- Your baby can maintain the calm alert state for long enough to feed.
- She has started licking and mouthing movements of her tongue.

Development

Premature babies develop according to their adjusted age, in other words the age they would be if they had been born on their due date. This is calculated as follows

Chronological age – weeks premature = adjusted developmental age

So a six-month-old who was born four weeks (one month) premature will have the development level of a typical five-month-old.

Until your baby is about two years old the adjusted age applies to everything, from feeding to sleep and development. When you read *Baby sense* (Faure & Richardson), read the chapter relevant to your baby's adjusted age.

If your baby was born very prematurely or she had many periods of medical instability or was at risk for brain damage or damage to her eyes or hearing, you will want to monitor her very carefully for about two years. If she is consistently not achieving target milestones for her adjusted age in each stage, bring it to the attention of your paediatrician.

The esSence of premature birth

- Premature labour (before 37 weeks) will be managed with a view to keeping your baby *in utero* as long as safely possible.
- If your baby is delivered before 37 weeks and requires support, you will need to adjust your expectations.
- Learn your baby's signals and communicate her state to her NICU team. In time you will know her best.
- Mimic the womb world with still touch, skin to skin care, quiet spaces and dim light in the NICU.
- Encourage early non-nutritive sucking and express early on.
- Breast milk, whether via breast or NG tube, is best for your prem baby's gut.

CHAPTER 17

1001 minutes

Read this chapter before birth

There will never be a moment like the moment you first hold your baby. In the haze of exhaustion you will touch his skin, smell his newborn smell and be overwhelmed with emotion. In the first 1001 minutes (about 17 hours) some things will be out of your hands, but knowledge is empowering and this chapter will guide you on giving your newborn the best possible start in life.

In an ideal world, your baby will be delivered healthy without medical interventions. In this case you and your partner can be actively involved and touch him as he enters the world.

- You may want to feel your baby's head emerging and will feel the wet, downy hair of your newborn for the first time.
- Your partner can deliver your baby to the world if he is keen to do so.
- Lay your baby on your tummy or chest, with the cord still pulsing, as he takes time to adjust to his new world, and takes his first breath.
- Delay clamping the cord for at least one minute. You or your partner may choose to cut it.
- If you are storing stem cells from the cord blood, the cord has to be cut sooner.
- Once the cord is cut, place your baby naked on your bare chest and cover him with a towel or blanket.

Having a C-section, for whatever reason, does not mean that you lose the opportunity for the same connection with your baby in the first few minutes. In general, you and your baby will be happier and calmer if together after birth and should not be separated unless it is necessary.

MOM SENSE

Looking back in months to come, you will be completely oblivious to what was happening with you in the hour after birth. You are likely to have been so enraptured with your newborn that you won't remember the procedures, stitches, injections and any other care.

Injections

You will receive a routine injection of oxytocin as your baby is born, to encourage delivery of the placenta and contraction of the uterus. This assists the natural contraction of the uterus, shearing off and expelling the placenta, and significantly reduces the risk of haemorrhage.

Stitches

If you have had a perineal tear or episiotomy you will need stitches to prevent bleeding and optimise closure and healing of the wound. The perineum is a very sensitive area and you will require local anaesthetic. The layers are usually stitched using an absorbable suture that will dissolve after a while and won't require removal.

C-section care

Following a C-section, your intravenous drip and catheter will remain in place for 12 to 24 hours. Once your spinal block or epidural wears off, you will require pain relief. Your anaesthetist will prescribe a combination of painkillers to provide maximal pain relief with minimal side effects. Most obstetricians allow mothers to eat and drink normally soon after C-section. You will be able to get out of bed about 12 hours after your surgery. You will feel pain or discomfort, but it should be manageable. The usual hospital stay following a C-section is three nights.

Bleeding

The placenta covered a large area of the uterus and this will now be a raw, bleeding surface. You will bleed vaginally whether delivery was vaginal or by C-section. The blood is initially bright red, and more than the blood loss normally experienced with menstruation. Blood can accumulate in the upper vagina and you may then pass an increased amount or clot when you stand up. You may also experience an increase with breast-feeding, which releases oxytocin and causes the uterus to contract.

Bleeding after delivery definitely calls for substantial maternity pads, and tampons must not be used. It's important to empty your bladder often in the day or two after birth as a full bladder can increase vaginal bleeding by preventing good contraction of your uterus.

BABY SENSE

Your baby's transition from the womb to the world is significant. Over the period of a few hours, he will move from complete dependence on you for the regulation of all his functions – temperature, heartbeat, hormones, emotions, sensory and nutritional – to having to manage many of these himself.

Apgar

The Apgar or newborn score is a measure of the wellness of your baby at birth, and is useful to establish if he needs intervention. It is observed at one minute and five minutes after delivery and your baby will get a score of two numbers (the one-minute number and the five-minute number).

As your baby is born, the opening between the two sides of the heart closes for the first time, directing blood to the lungs to become oxygenated, and your baby takes his first breath. This switch from foetal blood circulation to newborn blood circulation is absolutely amazing, and in the first few minutes your baby will be adjusting to all these changes.

By the time the cord stops pulsating after three to five minutes, your baby should be breathing well on his own and oxygenating his own blood via the lungs, with no further need for oxygen from your blood supply.

- A score of 9 at one minute is optimal (it's unusual to have a score of 10 at this time as your baby is still adjusting to life outside the womb so won't yet be completely pink).
- At one minute, any score of 7 or above is good, and your baby shouldn't require intervention and can stay on your tummy.
- A score of less than 7 means your baby will need some help, and the lower the score the more intervention and concern there will be.
- The score at five minutes tells you how your baby has responded to the intervention and whether any further intervention is needed.
- Most babies have a score of 9 or 10 after five minutes.

Procedures

With the aim of giving your baby uninterrupted time on your chest to warm up, adjust to our world, latch for the first time and initiate the natural release of oxytocin, you can request that no procedures are done for the first few hours, including weighing and measuring.

If you had a C-section, or a difficult vaginal delivery, a paediatrician will establish that your baby is well.

Your baby will have identity labels placed on an arm and a leg, possibly also on his back, in some hospitals. Your baby will be given a vitamin K injection soon after birth. This protects him against a fairly rare but very dangerous clotting disorder, which is difficult to diagnose until too late. An oral form of vitamin K is available, but is not as effective as the injection.

In some hospitals babies are routinely given antibiotic eye drops to protect them from neonatal ophthalmia (conjunctivitis), causing blindness if the mother is a carrier of gonorrhoea and chlamydia (common STDs). It is not necessary to give it to babies born by C-section, and in moms who have been screened and don't have these STDs. This eye ointment can cause irritation to your baby's eyes and blurred vision, which makes it harder for him to see you clearly after birth.

Sensory care

To help with the transition from the soothing, warm, dark, still world of the womb to the cool, clinical, light space of the labour ward, you can create a sensory womb space for your baby in the labour room:

TOUCH

- If your baby is born by C-section, warm the room to avoid the chill of a medical operating theatre.
- Stroke your baby.
- Help him to find your breast to latch on.

Skin-to-skin contact

Immediately after birth place your newborn baby naked on your chest – skin to skin. Cover the two of you with a blanket or towel to dry your baby and keep him warm (Kangaroo Care). Your chest temperature can miraculously increase or decrease by two degrees to regulate your baby's body temperature in a more intuitive way than an incubator. Aim to 'kangaroo' your baby for as many hours as possible in the early days. It is important to know that, if your baby is born healthy by C-section, he can be warmed up on your chest instead of being removed to a clinical incubator. While Dad's chest is unable to regulate temperature in quite the same way, the sensory effect of skin-to-skin touch with Dad is very helpful too.

Sound

- Speak to your baby in soft, soothing, slightly higher-pitched tones. He will recognise your and Dad's voices and your home language as his own.
- Play gentle music or white noise in the delivery room if it soothes you.

Sight

- Dim the lights and ensure that no lights shine in your baby's eyes – he has just emerged from a dark space and will be daunted by bright lights.
- Turn off all flashes for newborn photography if you can – use natural light.
- Make eye contact – your baby will keep looking around with tiny eye movements until his eyes rest on your eyes.
- Your baby can only focus 20–30 cm from his face. Hold him the distance of your forearm away so he can see your face.

Smell and taste

- You don't have to wash your baby after birth. Vernix is clean and moisturising for his skin. If he has a little bit of blood on him, wipe it off. Otherwise, you can leave him with the natural flavours and microbes of the womb space and birth canal.
- The familiar taste of amniotic fluid and vernix on his skin encourages him to suck on his hands. A drop of your hand-expressed colostrum on his mouth will help him become interested in feeding and to start rooting around to find your nipple.

Breast-feeding

Establishing breast-feeding is important and starts from birth. When welcoming your baby you can kiss and cuddle him and he may root around (opening his mouth and turning his head to touch on his cheek). Offer him your breast, so he can latch and feed.

Breast-crawl

If your baby is placed on your abdomen, he will make crawling movements with his limbs and bobbing up and down head movements, possibly finding your breast and latching unassisted after an average of 40 minutes. You can allow this process to happen naturally or assist your baby to latch.

Colostrum

Colostrum is the magic milk that your baby will feed on for the first three to four days until your milk has come in. It has the perfect combination of nutrients for a newborn and is packed with antibodies that line his gut and protect him from infection. It provides enough energy to keep your baby sucking and stimulating your supply until your milk comes in. It also acts as a laxative so your baby can pass the meconium stool.

Latching

It's important that your baby latches and suckles comfortably for you. An incorrect or shallow latch will quickly damage your nipples, which can make every feed really unpleasant. You may feel discomfort for the first few seconds, but if the pain continues beyond the first five seconds, particularly if it feels like the nipple is pinched or like sandpaper is rubbing on it, you need to take your baby off and relatch him. Ask for help with the latching if it's not comfortable.

A good latch has as much breast in the baby's mouth as possible (not just the nipple), particularly where the bottom lip is, as that's where the tongue is milking the breast. Your baby's mouth should be open wide.

How to latch
- Keep your hands off your baby's head, support his shoulders and neck and let his head lie back a little, so his chin comes in to the breast first, not his nose.
- Encourage him to open his mouth by teasing his lips – stroke them with your nipple. If that doesn't work, drop some milk into his mouth to show him what deliciousness is on the menu!
- It helps to make a sandwich with your offered breast, shaping it so it fits in the baby's mouth nicely.
- When tickling his mouth with your nipple, wait for your baby to open wide, and as he does, quickly bring him in to the breast so that he gets a good mouthful of breast.
- Hold breast and Baby close together for a few seconds until he gets into a good sucking rhythm, or relatch if he didn't manage to get a good latch or is pushing the breast away.
- If the latch looks wrong or feels sore, insert your clean pinkie finger into the side of his mouth to break the seal – don't just pull him off the nipple.
- Once he is sucking rhythmically you can slowly let go of the breast and bring that hand to rest on your other hand, making a circle of your arms, so you can relax your shoulders.

ROOMING IN
Having your baby sleep in your room in hospital and the early nights has been shown to increase the length of breast-feeding and chance of success with breast-feeding. So it is recommended that you request that your baby is not separated from you and has easy access to the breast when he needs to feed. If you are tired and need a few hours' respite, there is no harm in handing over care for a few hours while you sleep. Make it clear that your baby must be brought back to you when he needs a feed.

FEEDING
Your baby should latch and feed at the breast on demand – at least every four hours. Feeds need not take longer than 5 to 10 minutes per breast as the milk volumes in the first few days are small. There is no need to limit the feed times either unless it's painful, in which case you should be getting help to improve the latch.

Connecting
Bonding and attachment are two sides of a very important emotional process that you will go through with your baby. You will bond with your baby and your baby will attach to you. He needs to attach to you and his dad and form a meaningful relationship, as this is the foundation for future relationships.

However, before you feel immense pressure to make this happen, you also need to know that it is a very variable process. You may have fallen in love with your baby the day you knew you were pregnant or you may have been smitten from that first scan or when you felt him move. For some moms and dads, bonding does not happen in pregnancy but happens within moments of his birth. For other parents, it's a growth process that occurs over time in the first year.

How and when you bond is not critical – do not let yourself be consumed with guilt if it's not love at first sight. Consistent, loving parenting over the first 1001 days (three years) is vital and this awareness gives us time to fall in love.

HINTS FOR THE OTHER HALF

- Being present, physically and emotionally, at your baby's birth is the best experience in the world. You will love your partner in ways no one can prepare you for.
- Ask to be involved – cut the cord, touch his head or simply stand behind your partner's head and watch him being born, if the gore of seeing him emerge is too much. Make this birth your own too.
- Being at the birth, being caught up and actively involved in the drama of it, is a huge connector. So many women say, "I could not have done it alone". We long to be needed and feel important, and this is your moment!
- Hold your baby very soon after birth, if possible naked against your bare chest – not only will your baby love the skin-to-skin contact, but it will help release feel-good and love hormones in you too. This creates a magical moment that will be etched in your memory.
- Don't panic if you do not feel an immediate bond with your baby. In time you will fall in love.

The esSense of the first day

- You will be so captivated by your baby that you are unlikely to notice the oxytocin injection or stitches to your perineum should you need them.
- You will bleed a lot on the first day – bright-red blood that is heavier and redder than a normal menstrual cycle. Use sanitary pads, not tampons.
- Your baby will receive a vitamin K injection. Many other procedures are optional. Understand what is essential and what you would prefer to be delayed until after the first few hours.
- Kangaroo care is the best way to re-enact the womb world on a sensory level for your newborn.
- Guide your baby to the breast and latch soon after birth.
- Preferably have your baby sleep in your room from the start.

CHAPTER 18

1001 hours: The first six weeks

In the next 1001 hours – the first six weeks of your baby's life – you will be faced with a steep learning curve, one with the highs of falling in love and lows of feeling overwhelmed with the care of your tiny baby. This chapter will guide you on the physical element of your healing and your baby's early care. It is time to read *Baby sense* if you have not yet started the book.

Much of the first two days is filled with positive feelings and excitement as your family meet your new baby. And then comes day 3 … It's no myth that this is a tough day. Not only will you be preparing to go home if you didn't have a home birth, but your hormones also change and your milk comes in. Or you may wait with bated breath for the change and your milk doesn't come in. This may leave you worrying that you cannot meet your baby's needs.

Going home is always a big step and you may wonder how you can cope without the support of the nurses. Luckily most babies are calm in the first two weeks, easing us in gently.

MOM SENSE

After a nine-month period of gradual changes to your body, the first six weeks after birth will feel like a massive shift as your body heals from birth and attempts to return to normal (well, at least your new normal).

Bleeding

Bleeding continues for a surprisingly long time after delivery (three to six weeks). This discharge is referred to as lochia. Bleeding is initially bright red and heavier than with a period and blood clots may be passed when you stand. By the end of the first week, the volume will have reduced quite significantly and the colour will have changed to brown 'old blood'. The amount reduces to become more of a discoloured discharge (sometimes a little orange), which can niggle on until six weeks after delivery. Use sanitary pads (initially maternity ones) not tampons during this time.

CARE OF EPISIOTOMY OR PERINEAL TEAR

If you tore or had an episiotomy in natural childbirth, you will be sensitive in the vaginal area. Care of the area is for comfort as much as to aid healing and prevent infection:

- Place ice packs or a small plastic bag with frozen peas on the area, not directly on the skin, for 10 minutes and remove for 20 minutes.
- Stitches absorb so don't need removal, unless one is particularly tight and causing pain.
- In the first few days, when urinating, pour warm water from a jug between your legs into the toilet bowl, to prevent the burning sensation.
- Have a sitz bath, soaking the perineum in warm water with or without salt, for 20 minutes, three to four times a day, for relief. Use ¼ cup salt or this herbal recipe:
  - ½ cup Epsom salts
  - 2 tbsp baking powder
  - 2 tbsp witch hazel
  - 1 tbsp olive oil
  - 8 drops of lavender oil
  - 8 drops of camomile oil
- Slowly add ice cubes to the bath if the colder sensation is soothing. Pat dry gently.
- Fresh air on the wound (as often as is practical) is soothing.
- You will be more comfortable lying down than sitting and will need to find a soft and comfy chair for feeding, or feed lying down.
- Your doctor will prescribe anti-inflammatories for pain that are safe for breast-feeding.
- Anticipate the pain to intensify between days 5 and 7 – you may need more pain medication on these days.

Recovery from vaginal birth

Your body will recover on its own, at its own pace. Be patient with it. The uterus initially contracts, then involutes to return to virtually its previous size by six to seven weeks after delivery.

Your abdominal wall has been stretched and will take time to normalise and you may initially still look pregnant. While you will lose an incredible amount of weight in the first six weeks, most women have not achieved their pre-pregnancy weight, nor their pre-pregnancy waistline, by six weeks.

The vulva and vagina heal very well thanks to an excellent blood supply. Tears or episiotomies will be painful for the first 14 days and require painkillers. Small amounts of all medication will pass into the breast milk, but it is more important to alleviate pain and be able to cope with breast-feeding than to do without.

The increased elasticity in the vagina, allowing the stretching that occurs with delivery, facilitates its return to normal. You may have temporary lack of bladder control after vaginal delivery. This improves, so there is no need to panic in the first few weeks. Pelvic floor exercises (Kegel exercises) should be done regularly (see p. 109).

Recovery from C-section

Many of these points also apply to recovery from a C-section. Vaginal bleeding is similar. You will probably need regular pain medication for the first week. Thereafter you should be moving fairly easily but bending and twisting will still be uncomfortable and you will still need painkillers. Few women require them beyond two weeks. The scar will remain sensitive and tender for the first month (and will be tender to the deep kicks your baby gives into the lower abdomen for many more months). Make sure you have some full panties that don't irritate the scar area. Numbness around the scar is normal and takes several months to resolve.

WHEN TO CALL THE DOCTOR

Call your doctor if you experience:

Bleeding
- An increase in the heaviness of bleeding, especially a return to bright red blood after it has changed to brown or if you soak a maternity pad in an hour or less
- Still passing clots after two weeks
- The lochia (vaginal discharge after birth) smells unpleasant.

Infection
- Pain due to vaginal stitches increasing after seven days
- Redness or tenderness around a C-section wound, or oozing or bleeding from the wound
- Swelling, redness or pain in one area of the breast – could be mastitis or breast abscess
- Swelling, tenderness and redness of one leg – this might be a sign of thrombosis (a clot) and must be checked the same day.

Fever
- A temperature above 37,5 degrees, especially if associated with shivering and teeth chattering, is often a sign of mastitis (breast infection) or kidney infection.

Problems breathing
- Shortness of breath or chest pain could be signs of a pulmonary embolism (clot) and must be checked the same day.

Night sweats

You will find that you sweat a lot in the first few weeks after your baby is born. It's a hormonal response to help you get rid of the extra water you carried during pregnancy. It's common for breast-feeding moms to sweat for a prolonged time but it is almost always resolved by six weeks. Manage it with light cotton bedding and a clean set of cotton nightclothes to change into when you wake up in a sweat.

Sweating with a fever is not normal and is a sign of infection – have it checked.

Uterine pain when breast-feeding

When your baby suckles at the breast, oxytocin is released to help your milk flow. This hormone has an effect on the uterus – as it did in labour – and contracts your uterus, helping to reduce bleeding from the placental site and taking the uterus back to its normal size by six weeks. When this happens in the first three or four days post partum, as your milk starts to flow you may feel uterine cramps that can be quite painful and unpleasant. It's nothing to worry about.

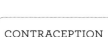

Your six-week check

You will have a post-partum check approximately six weeks after delivery. As well as serving as a reunion with your caregiver, this is to assess how you are coping physically and emotionally.

- Your doctor or midwife will enquire about any ongoing bleeding, or any pain related to stitches (vaginal or C-section).
- You should also be asked about bladder and bowel function.
- You will be examined (including a blood pressure check), and wounds will be checked.
- A cervical/pap smear is often taken.
- Contraception should be discussed, and issues such as sex and postnatal depression might be raised.

Getting back to your old self

You will never be the same – your body and mind are altered forever once your baby is born – but there are some activities that you will want to resume.

DRIVING

If you have had an uncomplicated vaginal birth, there is no need to postpone driving. If you delivered vaginally, but had a tear or an episiotomy, you can delay driving until it is comfortable to sit in a car, manoeuvre your legs and twist in the seat without discomfort. This may take a couple of weeks.

Following a C-section, you need to be able to sit comfortably wearing a seat belt, twist to look over your shoulder and move suddenly to use the pedals. Most women can do so by two to three weeks. Be sensible and delay driving if it is not comfortable.

EXERCISE

If you had a natural delivery, you can do aerobic exercise once you feel comfortable. That can be as soon as three weeks, once you are completely comfortable walking reasonable distances.

Following a C-section you can return to full exercise after six weeks, but this varies from one person to another.

CONTRACEPTION

Contraception will usually be discussed at your postnatal visit. For women who are exclusively breast feeding, falling pregnant during the first six months is unlikely but not impossible. Do not rely on breast-feeding as a form of contraception. If you are breast-feeding, oestrogen, and therefore the normal combined oral contraceptive (COC) pill, is contraindicated, as it reduces the supply of breast milk. Contraceptive options for breast-feeding women are either non-hormonal, or progesterone-only methods.

Non-hormonal methods include:
- Condoms
- The intrauterine contraceptive device (IUCD) (loop, coil or copper-T)

Progesterone-only methods include:
- The progesterone-only pill (POP) is a safe and popular option. It is not as effective in preventing pregnancy as the COC, and must be taken PRECISELY the same time (within three hours) every day.
- Injectable progesterones (Nuristerate or Depo Provera) are convenient and you don't have to remember them every day.
- The progesterone implant (Implanon).
- Mirena intrauterine system – a progesterone releasing IUCD.

- Going for a brisk walk with your baby will do an enormous amount of good for your head and your body.
- Kegel exercises are important.
- Join a class with fun, uncompetitive moms – the laughter and camaraderie will release those wonderful endorphins – just as important as the exercise itself.

INTERCOURSE

As the six-week mark comes around you anticipate many milestones, one of which is the expectation that your sex life can resume. However, you are suffering from lack of sleep, you may have little sexual desire, reduced vaginal lubrication, and you may not feel very sexy. Tender nether regions may make you both feel cautious. And of course you will inevitably be interrupted just as you get in the mood, if you manage to get that far!

Your partner needs to connect with you and feel close to you more than ever, so don't abandon your sex life. Oxytocin, which is associated with bonding and monogamy, is released in both of you during intercourse and is really important for your relationship. This hormone is also associated with breast-feeding, so your breasts may leak when you are aroused. Be matter-of-fact or laugh about it – it's part of the fun and games in a loving relationship. It may help to use some lubricant.

Resuming your sex life successfully is a combination of willingness on your part to engage, realistic expectations from your partner, not allowing resentments to build up, and a sense of humour.

BABY BASICS

Vaccinations in hospital

Before you leave the hospital your baby will be offered the BCG vaccine to protect against tuberculosis (TB), which is highly infectious. South Africa has one of the highest rates of TB worldwide.

The vaccine is given in the upper right arm by injection and will usually have no side effects until about five weeks later, when the site usually becomes inflamed and looks like a spider bite. This doesn't hurt or bother your baby and is no cause for concern. No treatment is required and the inflamed site should be left alone.

Most private hospitals also give oral polio drops, according to the South African schedule (EPI).

Cord

The plastic clamp on your baby's navel will probably be removed before you leave the hospital. The cord becomes black, looks like biltong, and falls off after 5–14 days.

You should clean the site once a day, more often if it is oozing or smelly. Clean it with a cotton ear bud dipped in surgical spirits, just at the insertion into the abdomen. Don't worry about the cord itself, as that is dry already. You could alternatively sprinkle Wecesin wound healing powder onto the site. Fold the nappy so that the cord stays above it and stays dry.

Once the cord detaches from the navel it usually oozes a browny-red skid mark on the vest, so continue cleaning it for another three to four days until it no longer requires attention.

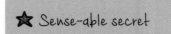

⭐ Sense-able secret
. . . .
When to worry about the cord
You should be concerned about infection if the base where the cord inserts into the navel is red, inflamed and hot.

Poo

Your baby's first stool is a thick, tarry, sticky green-black substance we call meconium. It can be hard to wipe off and putting Vaseline on her skin before she passes this stool can make it easier to clean.

By day four to five, soon after your milk comes in, the poo becomes light green and by day six or seven turns a yellow mustard colour, the consistency of Dijon mustard and grainy in appearance. Three to four poos a day from day seven will tell you that your baby is feeding well. The consistency can be quite loose, even runny.

Frequency varies considerably in breast-fed babies – from a poo every feed to only once a week once they are three to six weeks old. In formula-fed babies two poos a day or one every second day is normal.

If your baby's stools are not only infrequent but also difficult to pass, thicker than toothpaste or are like hardish putty or like pellets, your baby is constipated and you need to seek advice from your doctor or clinic sister.

Skin

After birth, your baby's skin is likely to become dry and flaky. Massage her with fragrance-free aqueous cream or natural vegetable-based oil. When cleaning the nappy area, you will find your baby has very sensitive skin. For the first few weeks use cotton wool and water or aqueous cream when changing her nappies. If your baby doesn't develop a rash or sensitivity, you can move on to wipes, which are much easier.

Milia

Your baby may develop pimply white spots mostly on her face, between four and ten weeks of age. This is usually a hormonal reaction. Don't fiddle or squeeze; usually no treatment is required.

Baby acne

From four to ten weeks your baby may develop teenage-like pimples on her face, neck and shoulders. This is as a result of the withdrawal of the maternal hormones. Don't fiddle or squeeze and no treatment is required.

Nappy rash

When your baby develops a nappy rash, a proper case of maternal guilt sets in as you wonder what you did or didn't do to cause her this irritation. Rest assured that many babies suffer from nappy rash, which is caused by ammonia in the urine and faeces burning the new soft skin of their bums. To avoid nappy rash:
- Change your baby's nappies frequently and clean the genital and anal area thoroughly at each change.
- Avoid perfumed or alcohol-based wipes – rather use cotton-wool swabs with cool boiled water until your baby is six weeks old.
- While good quality disposable nappies do not require the use of a barrier cream, you can use a preparation to prevent chafes. Milko balm is cheap and fragrance free.
- Make sure that cloth nappies are rinsed well.
- Leave your baby's nappy off at least once a day for a short period.

Treating nappy rash:
- If your baby has a mildly red bum, sprinkle some cornstarch (Maizena) into the nappy, which will dry the area well after each change.
- If the nappy rash persists, use a zinc-based antiseptic cream such as Sudocrem to soothe and treat it.
- Occasionally a nappy rash is more aggressive and spreads into the folds of your baby's thighs and develops raw lesions. This may be a rash caused by the fungus *candida albicans*. Ask your doctor or clinic sister to prescribe the right anti-fungal cream.

Jaundice

Mild jaundice (yellow skin) is visible in most newborns. Your baby's red blood-cells break down, producing bilirubin, which her liver is not yet able to process. If bilirubin levels are excessive, it turns your baby a little yellow. This often appears between days 3 and 5.

Jaundice is usually harmless and resolves over a period of a few weeks. Frequent breast-feeding in the first few days helps to decrease jaundice levels, as colostrum is an excellent laxative, speeding up the excretion of bilirubin.

If bilirubin levels are too high your baby will become drowsy and will not feed well, which exacerbates the problem. Bruising during birth, or blood type incompatibility between Mom and Baby, may increase the risk.

More severe jaundice is usually picked up before discharge from hospital but if you are already home and your baby is sleeping a lot and not feeding well and her skin appears very yellow in colour, particularly her eyes and the inside of her mouth, you need to talk to your doctor or clinic sister. If she considers it a problem she will do a heel-prick blood test. If the total serum bilirubin (TSB) is too high, your baby will be treated with phototherapy – placed under blue UV lights – as severe jaundice is dangerous if untreated.

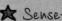 **Sense-able secret**

When to call your clinic sister or doctor

- In the first week home, it's not okay for your baby to sleep through the night. If your baby is too sleepy to feed, she needs to be seen by a doctor as this may indicate jaundice.
- If your baby doesn't have her usual energy and seems 'floppy'.
- If your baby is finding it difficult to breathe or breathing is laboured or grunty.
- If your baby has a fever, especially when she is less than six weeks old.
- If your baby is fussier than seems normal to you, and you are finding it difficult to get enough sleep or to calm her.
- If your baby has a rash you are worried about.
- If your baby is fussy during feeds.
- If you are worried your baby isn't growing or feeding well.

Bathing your baby

There is no need to bath your baby for the first few days – that newborn smell is delicious and, in addition to other benefits, vernix moisturises the skin. If your baby has blood on her hair or body that cannot be wiped off and it bothers you, it's absolutely fine to bath her as soon as you like. If there was meconium in the amniotic fluid, you will bath her, as it is irritating to the skin.

WHERE

Your baby can be bathed anywhere – the bathroom basin, in the bath with you, or in a baby bath. Make sure that the height is comfortable for you, because you need to take care of your back.

HOW TO BATH

First prepare the area by laying out the towel, nappy and clothes and then running a bath. Make it warmer than body temperature or your baby won't enjoy it – 36–38 degrees Celsius. Checking with a thermometer is not necessary.

Do not use any soap or shampoo. Using only water or aqueous cream for the first few weeks allows your baby's natural skin barrier to develop. Soap, preservatives and alcohol can disturb this process.

Prepare to wash your baby at her changing mat by washing her face first with water. Then take off her clothes and place her in the bath. Use a support to hold her or keep your non-dominant forearm under her back and hold her distant arm firmly while you rinse her off.

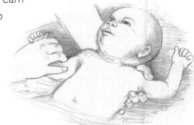

Most babies hate being dressed and undressed, so expect some unhappiness. You will probably be all fingers and thumbs the first few times, which can make it stressful.

GENITAL CLEANING

Your little girl's vagina is protected by her labia and is self-cleansing, so leave it alone. She may have a hormonal discharge on days 3 to 4 that can cause bleeding or a mucus similar to a period. Don't worry about that. Clean the labia front to back.

Your little boy's foreskin is not retractable for a number of years, so leave it alone, too.

TOP AND TAIL

Babies don't need to be bathed every day, especially in cold winter weather; a top and tail will suffice, unless they vomit (posset) a lot. To top and tail your baby, use clean, lukewarm water and cotton wool pads. Wipe her face with the damp cotton wool by cleaning her eyes separately, from midline outwards. Use another pad to wipe around her ears, mouth and neck. Using clean pads, wipe her bottom and the folds of her thighs too.

Feeding

After three to four days of feeding on colostrum, your baby will have stimulated your breasts sufficiently for mature milk to come in. When this happens, your breasts will be uncomfortably full. If you are very uncomfortable, ask your nurse or a lactation consultant to assist you with heat and cold packs and massage to relieve fullness. The engorgement can last for three days and frequent feeding in this time helps.

In the first few weeks you need to feed your baby on demand. Once your breast-feeding is well established and your baby is gaining weight well, feed her two- to four-hourly in the day (even if this means waking her to feed). Once she has regained her birth weight, leave her to wake you at night.

Your baby may demand feeds close together in the early part of the evening (cluster feeds) – encourage this if it is helps her to sleep for a slightly longer stretch later.

CIRCUMCISION

Circumcision is a controversial issue. There are few medical indications for performing the surgery, and it can be argued that we are born with a foreskin so why take it off? The procedure is painful, the wound can get infected and sometimes too much or too little foreskin is removed. Circumcision offers some protection from STDs and definitely reduces the risk of HIV infection.

It is a highly personal decision and mostly done for religious or cultural reasons. Circumcision is normally done in hospital between days 1 and 3, or on day 8 at a Jewish baby's bris.

If you are planning a circumcision, find an experienced surgeon. Local anaesthetic is used.

After the surgery, thorough hand-washing and good hygiene when changing nappies is recommended. Wipe Vaseline onto a gauze square and place over the penis to protect it from rubbing on the nappy. You can bath your boy the next day, using no soap, just aqueous cream, and let his penis soak in the water; no touching or cleaning of the penis is required. On day 3 to 5 you will see granulation tissue on the raw glans, which looks yellow, and this will slough off by day 5 or 6. By then the penis should be pink and healthy.

Seek medical help if there is active bleeding from the penis wound, any skin becomes black or your child becomes feverish or doesn't feed well.

★ Sense-able secret
. . . .
Burping your baby
Many babies bring up their winds on their own, while others need to be propped up with their back upright to allow the wind to escape. Deep stroking of the back or light tapping can help. It is not essential to chase every wind. If a wind has not come up by five minutes, it will come out the other end.

Weight gain

Your baby will lose up to 10 per cent of her birth weight in the first three to four days. By two weeks your baby should have regained her birth weight, a sign that feeding is going well. It is important not to get hung up on your baby's weight gain as a measure of her thriving or your success as a parent. Babies gain weight at different rates.

At this time, you can expect a weight gain of around 140–250 g per week. There may be times when her weekly gain can be as low as 100 g but if your baby gains less than 140 g for two weeks in a row, ask your clinic sister for advice on how to increase the weight gain.

You should visit your local well-baby clinic for weekly weigh-ins and chats with your clinic sister.

LOOKING AFTER YOURSELF

It is important that you look after yourself properly at this stage – drinking a lot of water, eating regularly and sleeping when you can.

Healthy eating

Eat a wide variety of foods to get the calories, vitamins, and minerals you need to remain healthy, according to your appetite. In general, mothers are hungrier during the first few months of breast-feeding, and you should not ignore feelings of hunger when producing milk for your baby. However, you do not need to eat for two – adding only an extra 500 calories per day is sufficient. This is the equivalent of 8–10 almonds, 125 ml full cream yoghurt, ¼ cup blueberries and ½ cup biltong.

It is not necessary to exclude any foods while breast-feeding – it is rarely your diet making your baby unsettled and exclusion diets simply limit food at a time when you should be eating a good variety. Focus on eating a well-balanced diet with plenty of green, leafy vegetables (these do not form gas), good quality protein, and, of course, plenty of water.

Enhancing milk production

- Drinking loads of water is the best way to enhance milk supply.
- Try a very diluted version of Jungle Juice, called Wonder Water.
- Drink a smoothie with good protein content.
- Medication such as Eglonyl and Maxolon can be used to increase milk supply; discuss this with your doctor or obstetrician

WONDER WATER

The high sugar content in Jungle Juice can aggravate candida (thrush). Rather drink Wonder Water. Make it by blending the following ingredients:

50 mℓ Schlehen Blackthorn Berry Elixir	1 sachet fruit-flavoured rehydration solution
3–4 ℓ water (or more)	A few drops of Rescue Remedy

SMOOTHIE

Blend the following ingredients and add 5 mℓ honey:

125 ml yoghurt	125 ml milk
4 strawberries	¼ cup blueberries
¼ tsp vanilla essence	2 scoops whey protein

BABY SENSE

If you have not read *Baby sense* by Meg Faure and Ann Richardson (Metz Press), it is time to do so. Here are five tips from this well-loved book:

MEDICAL INTERVENTIONS

Eglonyl is a prescribed medication used to treat depression and psychosis, with a side effect of increasing milk supply, which is a winning combination. It affects women differently and most women find it a huge help, to mood and milk supply. Since it crosses the blood–brain barrier and its effect on the baby's development is unknown, a knowledgeable doctor should prescribe it with caution. It shouldn't be used to treat a low mood, as there are more effective medications for this, but where a low mood and milk supply go together, it can be very effective at turning both around.

Maxolon, used to treat nausea, is also used to increase breast milk supply. There are no clear studies as to its effectiveness. Although the manufacturer can't claim safety in pregnancy and lactation, it is a frequently used treatment for nausea and vomiting in pregnancy and is recommended by respected authorities. Dystonic reaction, an abnormal movement disorder, is a rare side effect of Maxolon.

Motilium is another anti-nausea treatment used to increase breast milk supply. It is not registered for this use. While it is recommended by some, others warn against its use in pregnancy and breast-feeding.

Your baby has a sensitive sensory system

In general, your baby can cope with only short periods of limited stimulation. Just being alive in our busy world is enough stimulation for the average newborn. Do not focus on stimulating her senses at this age. Visual input in particular can be overwhelming, as babies battle to look away from something that is powerfully stimulating, like a ceiling light. In this period, only stimulate your baby when she is calm and alert – this will be a maximum of 10 minutes in an awake time period.

Mimic the womb world

Provide a fourth trimester of womb-like nurturing by looking to the womb world when creating a soothing space for your newborn.

TOUCH

Swaddle your baby. Swaddling mimics the womb world as your baby's immature little movements press against a boundary, much like the elastic walls of the uterus. The deep pressure of a tightly wrapped cotton swaddling blanket provides calming touch pressure and neutral warmth.

Since new babies are sensitive to being passed around, have close family members handle your baby in a quiet environment when she is content. Each time she is held by a new person, her sensory system takes in all the new sensory information about that person, especially their smell, touch and sounds.

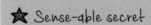 **Sense-able secret**

You may find that you are sensitive to your baby being handled too much. Listen to your gut and do not be shy to tell people that your little one has been passed around enough.

MOVEMENT

Carry your baby. Movement is lulling and soothing and most newborns crave to be close to their mom or dad. Do not worry about spoiling your baby in the early days. Use a sling or wrap carrier to create a womb space with deep pressure and the movement of your body.

SIGHT

Limit visual stimulation in the early days. While it is vital to stimulate the development of your baby's visual skills, visual input is very potent and can easily overstimulate your baby; therefore, time visual activities carefully. When your baby looks away from you or an activity, respect the time-out she requires and remove the stimulus.

SOUND

Play womb sounds to your baby. *In utero* your baby hears the white noise sounds of your heartbeat, the gushes of your blood and digestive sounds. Background white noise sound settles newborns in the early days.

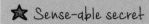
★ Sense-able secret

Signs of overstimulation
When your baby is becoming overwhelmed with the world, she will give you signals that she needs to sleep, needs less stimulation or needs a break from social interaction. These signs include:
- Bringing her hands to midline and trying to suck her hands
- Jerky and irregular movements of the arms and legs
- Grimacing and groaning
- Losing eye contact
- Extending her back and arching
- Hiccups and yawning
- Spitting up and reflux
- Blueness around the mouth or panting

SMELL

Do not wear any perfume, scent or aftershave lotion until your baby is a few months older; and then only introduce smells slowly and watch your baby's reactions. The smells of perfume and aftershave lotion can easily overload your baby. This is especially true when you're breast-feeding since your baby will then be in very close proximity to your bodily smells.

Sleep resets the sensory clock

Sleep is essential to learning, growth and being calm for newborns. Most newborns sleep for long stretches – almost from one feed to the next – until day 10 and thereafter may wake after one sleep cycle (45 minutes). This means that your baby will go from light sleep to deep sleep back into a light sleep state every 45 minutes and may then wake.

Regardless of how long your baby sleeps, watch how long she is awake and put her back to sleep after 50 minutes to an hour of awake time.

In the early days your newborn may have day and night muddled up, feeding more frequently at night and even being more wakeful when the rest of the world sleeps. We call this day-night reversal.

> **MANAGING DAY-NIGHT REVERSAL**
> - Differentiate day and night – make her room dark for sleep times, especially at night.
> - Keep night feeds very calm – no eye contact and don't even change her nappy if it is not soiled.
> - Spend time in the sunshine in the day while making sure your baby can't get sunburnt.
> - Swaddle your baby for sleeps.
> - Separate day and night with a bedtime routine.

Watch your baby's signals

Your baby will tell you when she is becoming overstimulated and moving into an active alert state.

CRYING AND OVERSTIMULATION

Between days 10 and 14 days your baby may begin to have periods of crying and pull up her legs, appearing to be in pain for prolonged periods, typically after the evening feed. You may be told your baby has colic or some digestive issue.

Evening crying is not usually related to digestive issues – it is due to the immaturity of the newborn brain. Your young baby's brain does not filter sensory information very well in the early days, which results in periods of overstimulation. Interacting and being awake in our world is stimulating for your new baby. By the end of a long day of interaction and stimulation, your baby becomes dysregulated and irritable.

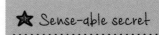 **Sense-able secret**

Preventing colic
Three quick tips to prevent colic:
- Regular day sleeps
- Reading your baby signals of overload
- Calming your baby's sensory environment

After a good feed in the evening, your baby will be hyper-responsive to internal sensory input (such as gas or feeling full) and will start to niggle. If you become anxious and try various soothing methods – rocking, jiggling, winding your baby – you may further overload a sensitive sensory system, resulting in further crying. Before you know it, you are faced with a three-hour crying spell.

For a more in-depth look at colic, read Chapter 8 of *Baby sense* (Faure & Richardson).

FUSSING AND CRYING

Babies all fuss, to some extent. Your baby will cry when she is hungry if two to three hours have passed since the last feed. Digestive issues do create discomfort in some babies. Your baby will cry if in pain or ill. Visit your doctor if unusual crying is accompanied by listlessness, lack of appetite, a fever or a rash.

YOUR EMOTIONS

It is common for a new mom to continue feeling anxious and emotional through the six-week postnatal period. Your hormones are settling and you are exhausted. If someone looks at you kindly you may feel the tears well up. This is not an indication that you are suffering from postnatal depression or even baby blues. At other times you are elated and utterly in love. This rollercoaster of emotions is very normal.

Is this postnatal depression?

It is essential to talk about it and to seek help, if you experience several of the following feelings:
- Feeling out of control, frustrated and very irritable
- The inability to think clearly, low concentration and forgetfulness
- That you are not the kind of mother you want to be
- Scared or panicky, anxious and worried, sad or miserable most of the time
- Resentful, oversensitive, unable to cope
- Unable to laugh or to feel joy
- Afraid to be alone and unusually tearful
- Feelings of shame or guilt and that your baby would be better off without you

- Feeling as though you are going crazy
- Fears that you may harm yourself or your baby

If you have experienced such distressing thoughts or feelings for more than 10 days, or you feel that things are getting worse, not better, seek help from your caregiver.

The most important thing to remember is that it is not your fault. You are not to blame. It is crucial that you tell someone you trust about these thoughts and feelings, and get the support and understanding you need and deserve. Your inability to cope with daily life is not the problem but may be a symptom of a real, treatable, medical condition. Seek support from the Postnatal Depression Support Association (www.pndsa.org.za).

Why am I not bonding?

The media paints a very romantic picture of a mom and baby deeply in love and enjoying every moment of falling in love. The reality may be far from this. Most moms have connected with and fallen in love with their baby at this point but some take a little more time. You may have a hard time falling in love or bonding if:
- you are significantly sleep deprived and feel unsupported in your role as mom;
- you are on painkillers and are feeling a little emotionally numb;
- your baby is a very fussy little one;
- your baby looks different from how you expected – especially in the case of a premature baby;
- you are battling with other distractions like financial concerns, illness or lack of safety in your home or marriage.

If this is the case for you, it is worth chatting to your doctor at the six-week visit or seeking help within your support system.

HINTS FOR THE OTHER HALF

- Your partner is beyond tired, overwhelmed and anxious at times and you will need to handle her with great sensitiviy. This time will pass but right now empathy is essential.
- You do need to watch for postnatal depression, which is often more evident through anxiety rather than despair.
- Sex is very important for you to reconnect but your partner may not feel sexy or up to connecting physically. A more subtle approach, starting with a back massage, may get you further than overtly pushing for intercourse.
- Make baby's bedtime routine your time – help with the bath, dressing and settling after the feed.
- Offer to walk your baby up and down the passage in a sling after the evening feed if she does not settle and is crying.
- Manage the practical elements of daily life – make sure that the car has petrol, the fridge has cabbage, milk, and all the essential basic fresh foods.
- Encourage Mom to call the lactation consultant if latching is tricky or she is struggling to relieve the engorgement. If you bought a breast pump and didn't wisely make friends with it before the birth, find it and work out how to use it so that you can help her to pump for a couple of minutes before latching, to soften very full breasts. Remind her that this was expected and will only last three days (or it may be wiser to let the lactation consultant say that!).

The esSense of the first six weeks

- You will experience significant bleeding that gradually reduces until it disappears by six weeks.

- You will have night sweats and have occasional pain in your uterus with breast-feeding. If your bleeding or pain is significant or you sweat with a fever, you need to see your doctor.

- Your baby will lose up to 10 per cent of her birth weight. This will be regained by two weeks as your baby feeds well and gains 140–250 g per week.

- Initially, feed your baby on demand. When your milk is established you can guide your baby to three- to four-hourly feeds during the day.

- Your baby may experience day-night sleep reversal – waking more at night than in the day. Provided she is gaining weight, do not offer a feed if less than two hours have passed since the last feed began.

- She should be sleeping for a large part of her day, 16 to 20 hours in a 24-hour cycle. Limit your baby's awake time to 45–60 minutes at a stretch and plan your caregiving and appropriate stimulation to take place within this time.

- You cannot spoil your newborn – this is a time when she may be niggly and settling her with holding and cuddling affirms her importance and helps her to learn to communicate her needs.

REFERENCES

Asbery K: *Altered Dreams: Living with Gender Disappointment*. AuthorHouse, 2008

Barham-Floreani, J: *Well Adjusted Babies*. Well Adjusted Pty Ltd, 2011

Bourquin I: *Practical Pregnancy, Birth and Early Parenting*. Pearson 2014

Cassidy T: *Birth Atlantic Monthly Press* 2007

Cuthlow T: *Zero to Five*. Pear Press 2014

Dewhurst's Textbook of Obstetrics and Gynaecology for Postgraduates 5th Edition. Blackwell Science Ltd 1995.

Eliot L: *What's going on in there*. Bantam Books 1999

Faure M, Megaw K, Strachan S: *Feeding Sense*. Metz Press 2010

Faure M & Richardson A: *Baby Sense*. Metz Press 2010

Gaskin, Ina May: *Birth Matters: A Midwife's Manifesto*. A Seven Stories Press 2011

Gaskin, Ina May: *Ina May's Guide to Childbirth*. Vermillion, London 2008

Haith M and Benson J (Eds) : *Encyclopaedia of Infant and early Childhood development* .Academic Press 2008

Lothian, J: *The purpose and power of pain in labour*. Guide to a Healthy Birth 2008

Lubbe W: *Prematurity – Adjusting your dream*. Little Steps 2008

Lukasse M, Vangen S, Oian P & Schei B: *Fear of childbirth, women's preference for cesarean section and childhood abuse: a longitudinal study* .Acta Obstetricia et Gynecologica Scandinavica 2010

Margulis J: *Your Baby. Your way*. Scribner 2013

Medina J: *Brain Rules for baby – How to raise a Smart and Happy child from zero to five*. Pear Press 2014

Murphy A: *The Seven Stages of Motherhood*. Pan Macmillan, 2005, 2010

Nelson-Piercy C: *Handbook of Obstetric Medicine 5th Edition* .CRC Press, 2015

NICE guidelines [CG62] Published date: March 2008 *Antenatal care for uncomplicated pregnancies*

NICE guidelines [CG62] Published date: March 2008 *Conditions and diseases, Fertility, pregnancy and childbirth*

NICE guidelines [CG190] Published date: December 2014 *Intrapartum care for healthy women and babies*

Otte T & Davidson G: *A Life begins – a parent's handbook*. Nestlé, 2010

Odent M: *Birth Reborn, What Birth Can and Should Be*. Souvenier Press 1984

Piotelli A: *Lecture on myths of pregnancy* GAIMH Conference 2015

Ratey J: *A User's guide to the brain*. Vintage Books, 2002

Rubin R: *Maternal tasks of pregnancy* Journal of Advanced Nursing Vol 1, Iss 5 p367-376, 1976

Sheldon R: *The Mama Bumba Way*. Findhorn Press, 2010

Shonkoff, JP, & Phillips, DA (Eds): *From Neurons to Neighborhoods: The Science of Early Childhood Development*. National Academies Press, 13 Nov 2000

Solomons J: *Hard Labour*. Cosmopolitan 2010

Sosa R, Kennell J, Klaus M et al: *The effect of a supportive companion on perinatal problems, length of labor, and mother-infant interaction*. N Engl J Med 303: 597, 1980

Stern D & Bruschweiler-Stern N: *The birth of mother*. Basic Books, 1998

Trethowan WH: *The couvade syndrome*. In Howell J (ed): *Modern Perspectives in Psycho-Obstetrics*. New York, Brunner & Mazel, 1972

Tsiaras A & Werth B: *From Conception to Birth: a Life Unfolds* Vermillion 2002

Welch, L, Miller, L: T*he Global Library of Women's Medicine* (ISSN: 1756-2228) 2008; DOI 10.3843/GLOWM.10415

Wilkinson C: *Dad*. Dad Books 2013

Wilson L & Peters T: *The Attachment Pregnancy*. Adams Media 2014

http://health.howstuffworks.com/pregnancy-and-parenting/pregnancy/issues/understanding-psychological-changes-during-pregnancy.htm

http://research.omicsgroup.org/index.php/Prenatal_development#Changes_by_weeks_of_gestation

https://umm.edu/health/medical/ency/articles/fetal-development

https://www.nlm.nih.gov/medlineplus/ency/article/002398.htm

www.pilatesnutritionist.com/prenatal-nutrition/

www.babycenter.co.uk

www.babycenter.com

www.evidencebasedbirth.com/waterbirth/

www.lowcarbdietitian.com/blog/guest-blog-post-is-it-safe-to-go-low-carb-during-pregnancy

www.motherinstinct.co.za

www.naturalhistorymag.com/features/142195/beyond-dna-epigenetics

www.nice.org.uk

www.nlm.nih.gov/medlineplus/ency/article/002398.htm - Fetal development

www.preggysense.com

www.pregnancysymptomsweekbyweek.org/

www.realfoodforgd.com

www.research.omicsgroup.org/index.php/Prenatal_development#Changes_by_weeks_of_gestation

www.umm.edu/health/medical/ency/articles/fetal-development

www.zerotothree.org

INDEX